HERBS — HOW TO GROW THEM AND HOW TO USE THEM

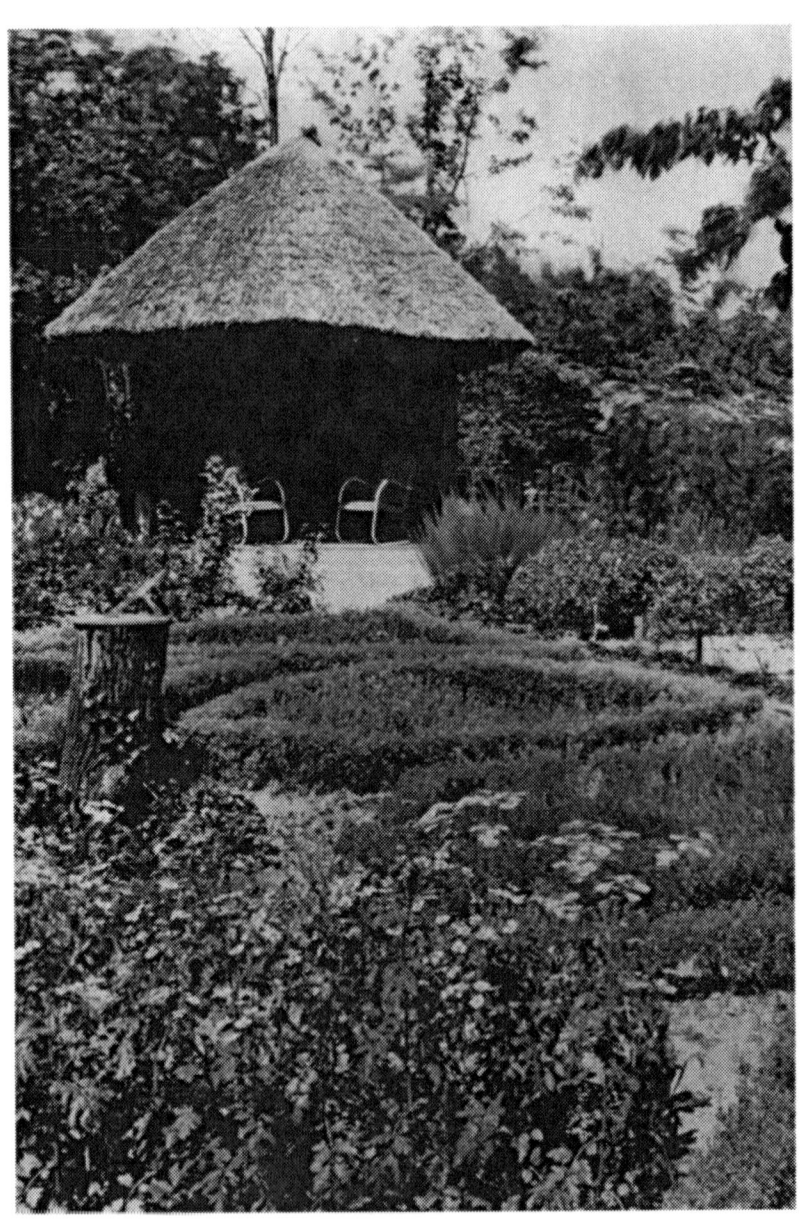

A LONG ISLAND HERB GARDEN
At the home of Mr. Clifford R. Beardsley, Huntington, Long Island, New York.

HERBS

How to Grow Them and How to Use Them

BY

HELEN NOYES WEBSTER

Illustrated

NEW EDITION, REVISED AND ENLARGED

BOSTON

RALPH T. HALE & COMPANY

PUBLISHERS

COPYRIGHT 1939, 1942, BY
THE MASSACHUSETTS HORTICULTURAL SOCIETY
First printing, January 1939
Second printing, December 1939

New edition, revised and enlarged
November 1942

PRINTED IN THE UNITED STATES OF AMERICA
BY THE ADAMS PRESS, INC., LEXINGTON, MASS.

DEDICATION

Since the first printing of a bulletin on herbs by the Massachusetts Horticultural Society, and nearly coincident with it, a small group of New England women with reverence for herbal wisdom of the past and belief in the present revival of herb gardens founded the Herb Society of America. To this Society, in recognition of its high standards, its ideals, its sincerity of purpose, and its untiring efforts to establish authoritative data concerning herbs, this book is dedicated.

ACKNOWLEDGMENTS

Since the pamphlet edition of "Herbs—How to Grow Them and How to Use Them," was issued in 1933, many friends and herb gardeners have contributed their experiences and helped me to make this a better book and to them my feeling of indebtedness is indeed sincere.

Nor could my task have been as pleasant without the encouragement of Mr. E. I. Farrington, who gave me generous assistance from his staff at all times.

From Dr. Elmer D. Merrill I have had the inestimable privilege of study in the Gray Herbarium. Mr. Stephen Hamblin of Harvard College has shared freely with me his field notes on herbs now growing in the Lexington Botanic Garden.

I am deeply appreciative of the help with the manuscript which my aunt, Miss M. E. Noyes, has given me, and grateful to my husband, Hollis Webster, for his criticism of the text and for his constructive suggestions.

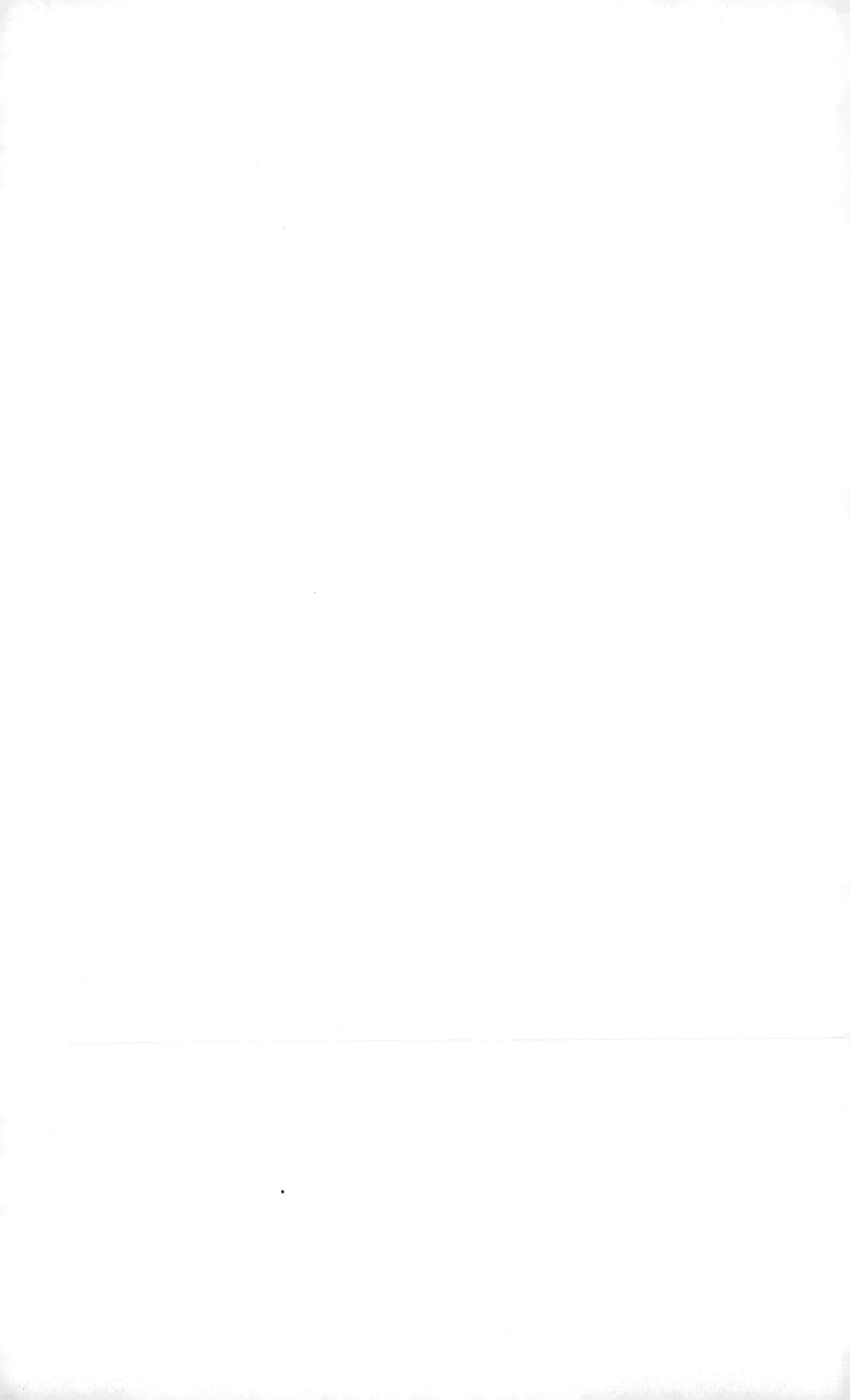

Contents

CHAPTER	PAGE
Foreword	13
I. Early Periods and Designs of the Herb Garden	17
II. Colonial Gardens	47
III. A Garden of Wild Herbs	62
IV. A Few Important Herb Families and Their Genera	71
V. Doctrine of Signatures	79
VI. Medicinal Herbs	81
VII. General Horticultural Directions for Herb Gardens	88
VIII. Commercial Growing of Herbs	104
IX. Drying and Curing Herbs	106
X. Uses of an Herb Garden	109

XI. Herbs as a Cottage Industry	118
XII. Cooking With Herbs	120
XIII. Check List of Herbs for Modern Gardens	141
Bibliography	187
Index	193

List of Illustrations

A Long Island Herb Garden	*Frontis.*
Garden to Farmhouse of 1861 with Bee Garden Adjoining the house	19
"Ringing Bees"	21
Bee-House with Magpie in Cage	21
Empress Komyo (710-793 A.D.) Gathering Herbs for the Sick	28
Seventeenth Century Still-House	Facing page 32
Bee Garden 17th Century	Facing page 32
Herb Garden at Storrowtown	Facing page 33
General Design for the Storrowtown Herb Garden	Facing page 33
The King's Herb Woman, Miss Fellowes, and Her Maids, 1821	37
Divers Forms or Plots for Gardens	39
Burnet (Pencil drawing by Louise Mansfield)	46
Formal Herb Garden of Pardee Morris House	Facing page 48
Experimental Plot of Sage—Variety "Holt's Mammoth"	Facing page 48
Rosemary at Entrance Gate	Facing page 49
Walled Herb Garden	Facing page 49
Chrysanthemum cineriaefolium Pyrethrum	72
Hedeoma pulegioides American Pennyroyal	74
Entrance Planting of Herbs, Weathered Oak Herb Farm	Facing page 80
Path Planting of Sweet Herbs	Facing page 80

LIST OF ILLUSTRATIONS

"Apothecary Shop" of the North American Indian Medicine Man . . . . Facing page 81
Rosemary, Tall Mugwort and Chives . . . Facing page 81
Hyocymus niger Henbane 82
Panax quinquifolium Ginseng 84
Pennyroyal 86
Mandragora autumnalis Mandrake 87
Origanum Dictamnus L. "Dittany of Crete" 94
Dentate Lavender 96
"Time Ambles Withal" . . . . Facing page 96
Dipping Well in an Herb Garden . . . . Facing page 96
Doorstep Planting of Herbs . . . . . . Facing page 97
Cultivation of Herbs at the Lowthrope Landscape School . . . . Facing page 97
Spike Lavender 98
Pinnate Lavender 101
Dioscorides receiving the root of the Mandrake from the Goddess of Discovery 102
The Great Ocimum; Sweet Basil 132
The Small Ocimum; Bush Basil 132
Spearmint, *M. spicata* 163
Watermint, *M. aquatica* 163
Wild Mint, *M. longifolia* 164
Woolly Mint, *M. rotundifolia* 164
Cornmint, *M. arvensis* 165

FOREWORD

With the revival of interest in the old herb gardens of our forefathers we need some compilation of scattered bits of information about the culture of herbs and their uses in cookery and medicine, as well as of the folklore, superstitions and legends connected with them, for every country today has forgotten much of the herb lore which had accumulated with its growth and that of its people.

The ancient classification of all plants into herbs, shrubs and trees is not without complications for, as we all know, there is overlapping of these groups. Shrubs and trees are woody; so is the herb rosemary; so also are some of the thymes, southernwood and English lavender. The shrub, privet, and the tree, willow, with much more wood of secondary growth, have herbal significance. Elder, a good old herb in English parlance, is a shrub because of its wood and dimensions, as also is box, another useful herb of antiquity.

Botanically the term *herb** has come to signify plants more or less tender, even if slightly woody. As annuals they die out completely at the end of the first season and must be reproduced from seed. Such are the tender herbs, dill, ambrosia and sweet mugwort.

Garden sage, hyssop and rue are sturdy, woody, perennial herbs which persist from year to year. The medicinal herbs, foxglove and Canterbury bells, or throatwort, are typical biennials with a life span of two years, at the end of which time a new generation must spring from seed. Angelica, parsley and others may have their natural biennial existence prolonged a year or more by cutting all seeding stems.

Famous old herbals concede to every plant its virtues and describe several hundred species of flowering plants which would not be considered at all today, by popular conception,

---

*In speaking the word *herb*, Englishmen nowadays tend to keep the h whereas Americans generally drop it. See Webster's Dictionary.

as herbs. Popularly, we have accustomed ourselves to using the term *herb* as that of a fragrant plant with medicinal or culinary use; nor is size any criterion, for the wee Corsican mint is as noble an herb as the lusty seven-foot lovage. Therefore the Herb Society of America has chosen to define an herb as "any plant that may be used for pleasure, fragrance, or physic."

The medicinal plants, whether of field or garden, are sometimes referred to as *simples* because each was supposed to hold within its power a simple remedial virtue for a simple ill.

The list of these *physic herbs* is long. Nearly four hundred years before Christ was born, Theophrastus, a pupil of Aristotle, studied in the herb garden of his teacher well over three hundred simples and wrote about them. Four centuries later, the great Greek physician, Dioscorides, wrote his herbal and, for a thousand years after, doctors the known world over prescribed these herbal remedies and effected cures by them.

One phase of changing economic conditions in every country during these World Wars is a revival of practical interest in the therapeutic value of the simple healing herbs, and notwithstanding the skill of the modern chemist in compounding synthetic remedies, many of these plants are used by physicians today. Because aconite and foxglove have become perennial border favorites does not mean that they have lost their therapeutic value, nor have the rose, violet, valley lily, squill, mallow and many others.

With the stabilization of the imports during the brief period before European hostilities again upset the economic world, drug and condiment herbs, including digitalis, hyocymus, valerian, chamomile, coriander, thyme, marjoram, pyrethrum, could be grown abroad with less labor cost than here in the United States. Now (1942) the scarcity of these herbs is being felt, and particularly in the medical world is it a matter of vital importance. Consequently in connection with the great laboratories and drug and spice concerns, there is a renewed interest in the commercial growing of the more important herbs. That experiments will lead to the industrial permanency now seems likely.

The old term *worts*[*] is still used for herbs in isolated regions in the Virginias and Carolinas where the spoken English still savors of Anglo-Saxon purity. The term however is not used in its original meaning which was root or plant, but seems to be applied particularly to herbs having specific uses whose prefix designates the use. For example the herb mugwort was used in brewing; pewterwort was a scouring herb; prick-songwort was an old name for honesty because its round, silvery disks resembled the notes called "prick-songs" on Elizabethan music sheets.

Yarbs is another loved and homely name, and the "yarb patch" by the humble Colonial dwelling included those precious simples yarrow, tansy, Bouncing Bet and rampion. To be sure we of today call them weeds of the wayside and the rubbish pile, but by right of ancient lineage, in service to mankind, yarb aristocrats they remain.

Sweet herbs are those of aromatic fame with odoriferous, pungent leaves and flowers. Their distilled oils used in perfumes and having other industrial uses are of great importance. Rosemary, lavender, sweet marjoram, thyme, sage, savory, anise, fennel and basil are among the sweet herbs.

Pot herbs are succulent, leafy vegetables and roots which add once unsuspected value to the boiling pot of "spring greens." As "salad herbs" they are eaten raw, but the line between these herbs and herbs in other groups is not sharply drawn. Chives, parsley, tarragon and chervil are admitted here. In old nursery lists are found intriguing names of pot herbs long since forgotten — blitum, Good King Henry, skirrets, roquette — which pique the curiosity of some of us who still limit the terms "pot" and "salad" herbs to lettuce, dandelions and spinach.

---

[*] See *The Herbarist*, 1935, Publication Herb Society of America, "A List for an Old English Wort Garden," Ella S. Greenslet.

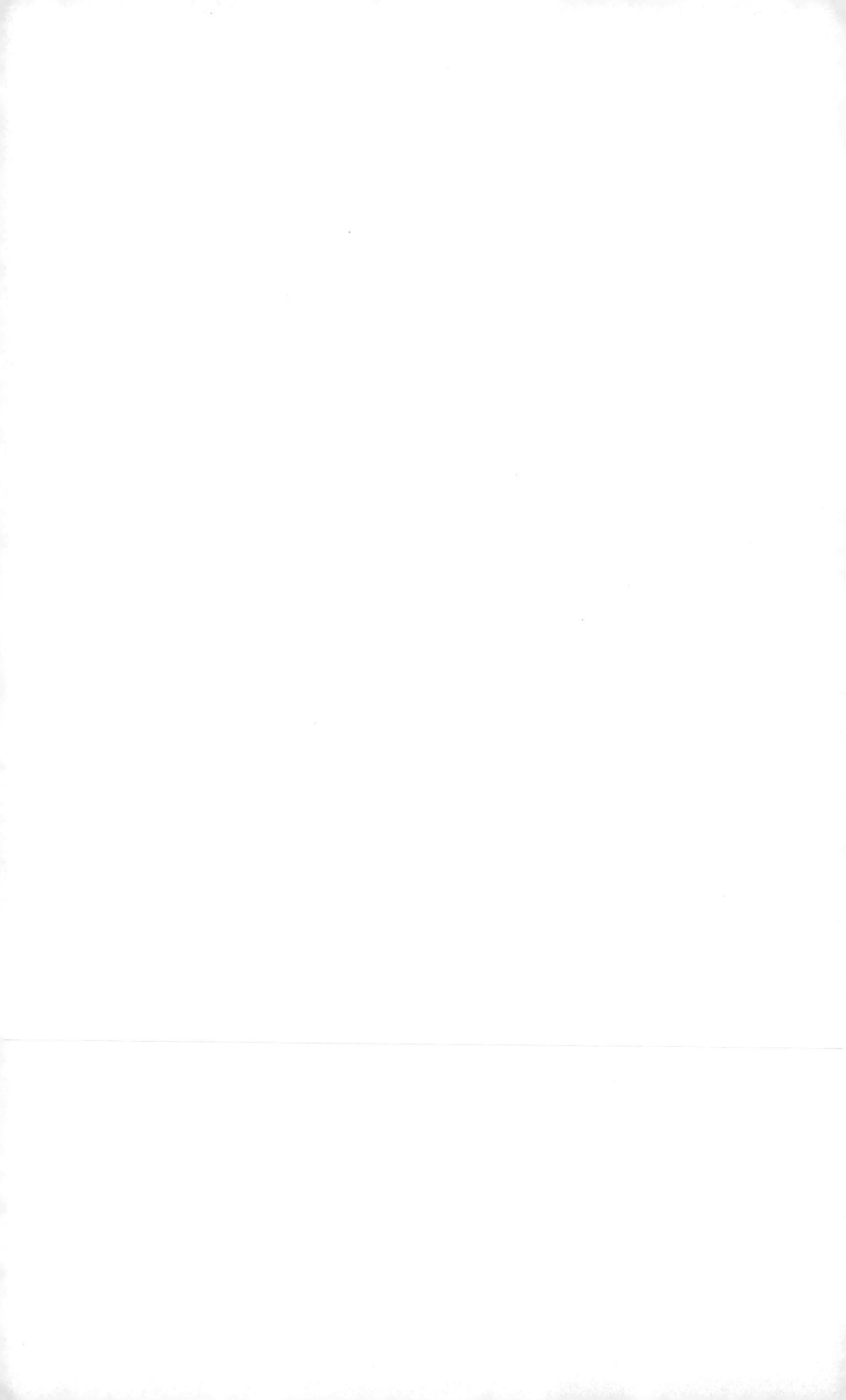

CHAPTER I

EARLY PERIODS AND DESIGNS OF THE HERB GARDEN

IT WOULD be indeed presumptuous to dictate to any lover of herbs the form his garden should take. Collecting simples for any type of garden is always an individual and zestful pursuit comparable to no other and there are many garden patterns in which to place them.*

Therefore the following are merely suggestions on which the reader may care to formulate some plan of his own.

If he is sympathetic to the close relationship between period architecture and its contemporary gardens he will be led into alluring hours of research. From ancient manuscripts and herbals, plant lists of historic gardens from all parts of the world, and the innumerable "Medical Botanies" published in the early years of the last century the herb gardener draws inspiring information. Adventure in itself is the study of flower and garden settings in the famous wall and canvas paintings of the old world and the interpretations of legends woven into the colorful Jacobean tapestries in museum and art galleries.

If, also, the herb gardener collects the facts and fancies connected with his plants, unusual superstitions, legends and uses, and verifies their authenticity, he helps to preserve a wealth of material before, in our modern rushing days, all is lost in the oblivion of a less exciting past. Here let it be emphasized that no detail is too trivial or homely if it adds to the knowledge and understanding of the tremendously important part that herbs and their uses have played in the lives of all peoples.

---

*See *The Herbarist*, 1935, Publication Herb Society of America, "Designs for the Herb Garden," Frances T. Norton.

Never in reality can the wondrous gardens of the East be made to live again, but in the "Song of Solomon" their trees, living waters and fragrance are still garden music.

Every herb gardener should read the beautiful descriptions of these gardens which Miss Eleanour Rohde has given us in several of her delightful books.

As we read the classics, we are amazed to find how little of the gardening that Roman horticulturists knew so well is new to us today. Scholarly research reveals that almost every plant and shrub and tree found in the Virgil garden have some herb interest and are available now for use in a reproduction of that classic plot. The maker of such a garden must love the beautiful poetry of the Bucolics and Georgics in which the poet writes with lyric accuracy of his herbs and bees.

Bee Gardens

Reminiscent of the classic era in garden history, is the modern interpretation of the bee garden.* Inspired by very early treatises of Greek authors, the modern architect of such a garden connects the bee garden with the herb garden itself.

This little out-of-doors bee room, perhaps the home of two or three hives of bees, may call to mind the tiny mediæval "Hortus Inclusus." But equally charming, fragrant and musical is the bee garden of larger size, designed for beauty, "honey herbs," and good methods of modern bee keeping. Cedars intertwined with roses and honeysuckle make enclosing walls not too high, for the room must not be hot and airless. Opposite doorways are cut in the hedge to let in the breezes and give passage into the herb garden beyond.

To fill the combs with a rich blending of all herb flavors, there bloom in that herb garden and its hedges, the season through, nectar-bearing flowers recorded in bee literature for two thousand years.

---

*See *The Herbarist*, 1936, Publication Herb Society of America, "Old Bee Literature," Ella S. Greenslet. Also *The Herbarist*, 1937, "Bee-Lore," Martha G. Stearns.

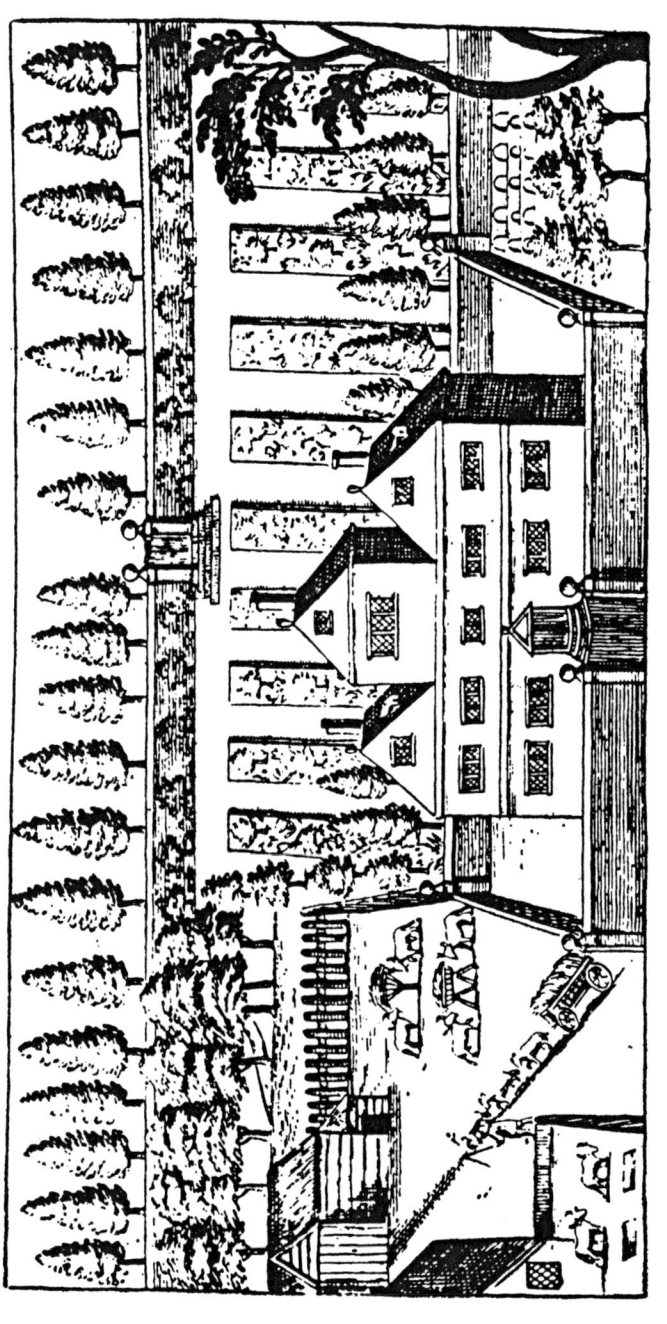

GARDEN TO FARMHOUSE OF 1681, WITH BEE GARDEN ADJOINING THE HOUSE

*Taken from Worlidge J. Systema Agriculturae, The Mystery of Husbandry Discovered, London, 1681, 3rd Edition.
Courtesy Publication Committee, Herb Society of America*

"All about let there be luxuriant growth of green Cassia and wild Thyme with its spreading perfume and abundance of strongly scented Savory." (Georgics, Book IV.)

Bee keeping has been associated with herb gardens since time immemorial. Plant spice bush and shad bush, teasles and thistles in the hedgerow, also button bush and chicory. If in the garden itself you will not grow the weedy milkweeds, although to the bee they are the sweetest of forage herbs, you will include in your perennial border a few plants of butterfly weed or pleurisy root, as the Colonists called this orange milkweed, and always the fennel giant hyssop *Agastache foeniculum*. Thymes of many kinds will last the season through. Over the white beds of the little earth-clinging white thyme, all day the bees hover happily, scarce lifting their wings as they drift from flower to flower. And the gardener stands, eyes half closed, every sense tingling to the ecstasy of that musical mist.

The hives in this modern bee room must be modern, but painted in soft pastel shades they harmonize with the garden and are not unpicturesque. The conical braided straw skep or the slab hive of mediæval Europe may be nearby for interest or historic accent.

But the bees, like the herbs they suck, are descendants of the same golden strain that lived with the mythical gods on Olympus, and although we have learned much of modern beekeeping methods we have never changed that music of the hive and its cadence, noted in scale and clef centuries ago.

Somewhere in the background must be willows, for from the golden pollen of their catkins comes the first beebread of the early brood in the hive. In the hedges plant all manner of early bulbs — squills, crocus, snowdrop and the winter's aconite. If you do not think of these as herbs read sixteenth-century Gerarde and Parkinson.

Rosemary must live through New England winters indoors, but in the early spring days set it in the bee garden — lots and lots of it.

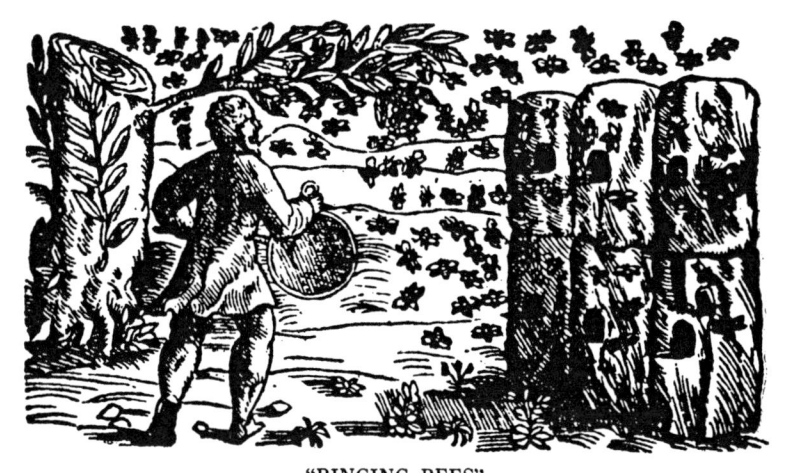

"RINGING BEES"
*From Matthiolus Commentarii in libros sex Pedacii Dioscoroidis
Venetiis, In Officina Valgrisiana, 1560*

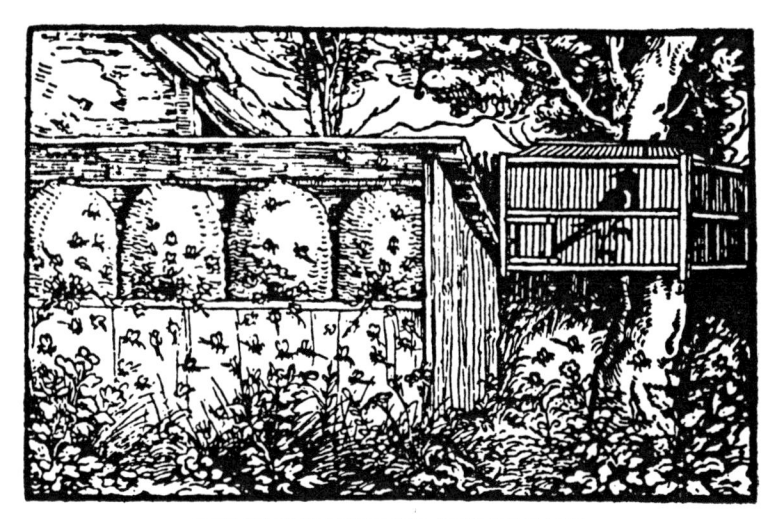

BEE-HOUSE WITH MAGPIE IN CAGE
*Woodcut by Hans Heiditz—German translation of Crescentius,
Frankfort, 1583
Courtesy Herb Society of America*

"As for Rosemarine, I lett it runne all over my garden walls, not onlie because my bees love it, but because it is the herb sacred to remembrance, and therefore, to friendship, whence a sprig of it hath a dumb language." (Sir Thomas More.)

All through the summer, the bees are delirious with joy over the ever renewed nectar in the procession of blossoming herbs, basils, lavender, roses, anchusa, borage and early cresses. They hover above the opening buds of ground ivy until some morning they find the ground covered with a sheet of its blue flowers. With this herb the serious business of nectar gathering starts. Let the bee keeper grow hyssop, germander, catnip and all kinds of mints, wild marjoram and savory, lemon balm and bee balm. Plant clover and thymes in the turf and scatter sweet meliotus freely outside with buckwheat and sanfoin.*

Mediæval Gardens

To reproduce a mediæval garden of that mysterious and fascinating period in English history between the late ninth and fourteenth centuries, absolute accuracy must yield to imagination and fancy, for of those and earlier years slight record remains.

Few manuscript herbals escaped the destruction of the Dark Ages. What information we have is given us in Druidical reference and in the Anglo-Saxon Leech Books, one of which was known to Alfred the Great. Our most authentic information of that period comes from the rare manuscript herbals transcribed by the monks in the comparative security of the monastery.

The Druids, Celtic priests of ancient Gaul and Britain, healed by the herbs' magical power over human beings and by incantations said over the simples as they were gathered. Herbs which guarded the well against evil were many. We

---

*See "Herbs for Bee Gardens," Stephen Hamblin, leaflet of Lexington Botanic Garden, April, 1942.

EARLY PERIODS AND DESIGNS OF THE HERB GARDEN   23

read of henbane, primrose, club moss, the sacred verbena, mistletoe and anemone (probably pulsatilla).

In Anglo-Saxon literature there is frequent reference to betony, mugwort, yarrow, feverfew, pennyroyal and sage; but the Saxons, so Mrs. Grieves, the great English herbalist of today, tells us, used all those herbs which the early Romans of Caesar's legions brought to Britain. They include lupine, nettles, coriander, rosemary, borage, iris, southernwood, onion, fennel, hyssop, rue, chervil, chives, celandine and many more.

Monks and nuns in the monastery gardens grew medicinal and cooking herbs and recorded with great care facts about their culture and uses.

We read that early in the history of the Christian church the cultivation of herbs was forbidden because of the pagan rites connected with their usage. But after endowing the lily, the violet, and the rose with divine symbolism, these plants were received again into the monastery gardens and grown with the healing herbs. Heartsease was dedicated to the Trinity, the lily signified purity of the soul, and the rose the red blood of the martyr.

If lured into reading "Mediæval Gardens" by the English scholar, Sir Frank Crisp, the reader will be tempted to create a Charlemagne garden.

That celebrated king, Charles the Great, died in 814 A.D., but the imprint of his imperial herb gardens throughout central Europe remains. The story is told how the learned monk Alcuin came by royal command from Ireland to teach this enterprising and progressive king all that he knew of herbs and their uses. It is said that the first "Question and Answer Primer" grew out of these lessons.

Said Alcuin to Charlemagne: "What is an herb?"

Answered Charlemagne: "The friend of the physician and the praise of cooks." This answer has not lost its savor today.

The king's wish that anise and fennel be grown near every dwelling accounts for their widespread distribution in Europe.

With similar purpose American "Johnny Appleseed" in 1805 scattered fennel seed along his hedgerows.

Perhaps these tiny mediæval gardens, close within the confines of monastery, castle and palace wall, were the beginnings of the great seventeenth-century Physic Gardens wherein were collected medicinal herbs from all the known world. The monks were the healers of body as well as soul, and ministered with equal skill to the rich and poor alike.

In their kitchens were distilled and concocted potions for their sick and cordials which are still famous for their blended herb flavors. Benedictine, for instance, a favorite cordial, to quote the International Encyclopedia, "was originally manufactured by the Benedictine monks, though since the French Revolution its manufacture, now a trade secret, has been controlled by a commercial company. It is believed that the volatile constituents of cardamon seeds, arnica flowers, angelica root, lemon peel, thyme, nutmegs, cassia, hyssop, peppermint and cloves enter into its composition." The small glasses in which this and similar cordials are served are said to represent the medicine glass in which the potion was given to patients.

A description of the ninth-century monastery of St. Gall in Switzerland and a pattern of the herb garden itself show the small, symmetrical, raised beds with each herb in a plot to itself.

In connection with the palaces of later mediæval years, the gardens became more elaborate. But the rambling garden of later centuries was unknown in the Middle Ages. Compared to the variety of later day flowers, the simples were few, but how rich in fragrance, symbolism and living beauty those gardens must have been! Gardens of this period were always enclosed with brick, stone, hedges, wattled fences, or the picturesque walls of mud and straw. In the latter part of the period beautifully wrought iron work appeared.

The mud-walled monastery garden is seen again in the cottage gardens of Devonshire, gardens which the centuries have so little changed. Let the wayfarer pause in some narrow Devon lane and, head uplifted, sniff the rosemary, which, growing up from within, falls over the wall to his head. A narrow gate at one corner invites entrance and admits into the sweet garden enclosed. Inside, the hard-baked mud walls are bound with jessamine and lavender, rosemary and honeysuckle, and there are bronze and gold wallflowers in every crevice. An ancient straw skep, home of the bees, must be in some sunny corner; and even though empty, it should remain.

To whom this experience falls comes the vision of making for himself one of those lovely old Devonshire gardens so curiously unchanged since Anglo-Saxon days.

It is a pretty fancy of today to make a garden of this pattern in an abandoned cellar hole where lavender falls over the stones and sunlight sifts through gnarled old apple trees above the herbs.

A clever modern gardener used the long withe-like stems of living viburnum bushes to make a wattled fence around her potting shed. These fences which we observe so frequently in early paintings look sturdy and picturesque, and seem to have been made by weaving flexible branches around upright posts. Probably cornel, osiers (willows), hornbeam and hazel were used.

The Hortus Inclusus, a mediæval feature in gardens was a tiny garden entirely hedged or fenced within a larger one, and may have been a place for quiet meditation, for it was planted only with turf.

Movable garden furniture as we know it does not appear until after the mediæval years. Exedrae were the high-backed stone seats of classic times. Turf seats were built sometimes into the surrounding walls of the garden. If not a part of the wall, these seats were mounds of earth faced with brick, stone, or wattled fencing. The surface top was turfed or planted with sweet-smelling herbs, which grew into a thick, close-cropped mat. Chamomile was used thus, thyme, and even mints, though which species of mints were low growing enough for this purpose I cannot imagine. A canvas primitive shows a Mary garden, the Virgin seated on the turf seat which is made around a single tree. All herbs in reproduced Mary gardens should be symbolical in name or legend of the Virgin. In reproducing the mediæval garden today these turf seats may be ingeniously introduced into corners or along an inner wall. Of course if the mound surrounds a tree the encircled trunk must be "welled" to keep the earth from the bark.

One of the loveliest features of those gardens was the fountain. It appears in almost every picture and, as the period progresses, these fountains grow in beauty of design and elaboration. Water was always introduced in some way into the mediæval gardens, perhaps as a tiny stream, the bathing pool, a dripping sluice or the dipping well.

We are adapting to the really beautiful church architecture of today the cloister gardens of the Middle Ages. As in those days, they are peaceful places enclosed by covered pergola, cloister columns, or walls of the cathedral itself. In them the flowers of the church, iris, roses, lilies and violas, seem particularly at home, with other herbs of healing. Here against cool, shaded walls nepeta, ground ivy and periwinkle thrive with box and true myrtle.

The mint pool belongs to the ninth century and before. It may be properly a part of a cloister garden. Somewhere I have seen a curious old wall picture of this interesting feature. As I remember it, an old monk, with robes tucked under his girdle, bends stiffly over his garden of mints which seem to be of many kinds. In the distance we recognize tall angelica or it may be lovage, but this rocky pool seems to be in a low, disused, unornamented part of the garden — just where we would expect the mints to grow. Through a crude sluice of hollowed log, which looks moss-grown and slimy, the water is dripping from somewhere into a shallow and mud-bound pool. "Along with man's beginning grew the Mints, and they came to be dearly loved by the church for their fresh, vigorous fragrance and omnipresent usefulness."

Among reproductions of mediæval gardens, the cloister garden in Fort Tryon Park, New York, is unique. It is connected with the Metropolitan Museum of Art. In ideally happy setting, this garden is true to period in form as well as are the herbs grown therein.

There are definite possibilities for adapting cool, green, cloister gardens to the diminutive, high-walled city yard. Periwinkle, ivy, and Gill-over-the-ground are smoke-resistant, and spring bulbs have their own lovely way of breaking through the spring greenness of these herbs. Rosemary and myrtle, the true *Myrtis communis,* must be grown in tubs of good sandy loam. Sweet geraniums and lemon verbena, though introduced into England at much later dates, do not seem out of place among the truly mediæval herbs. All have to come indoors out of the cold winters. Thymes will live for a season or two in the city garden, but they love too well pure air and unfiltered sunlight. Mints are a joy, for, given a rich pocket of soil to their liking, they will thrive under the drip of a hidden wall faucet.

Medicinal and Other Herbs Known in Mediaeval England
(Sixth to Fifteenth Centuries)

The herbs included in the following list are chosen because of their interest and adaptability to New England gardens. The complete list is published in Crisp's "Mediæval Gardens," taken from MSS. Sloane, 1201, in the British Museum.

ACONITE, *Aconitum napellus*—Showy herb with dark blue flowers. Roots poisonous if eaten.

ALKANET, *Anchusa officinalis*

AMBROSIA, *Chenopodium botrys*

ANISE, *Pimpinella anisum*

BASIL, *Ocimum basilicum*—Several varieties.

BETONY, *Stachys lanata*—This species is the perennial *woolly betony,* with large, very woolly gray leaves. The species known and used in Anglo-Saxon and mediæval therapy is *wood betony (Betonica officinalis* or *Stachys officinalis).* These two herbs belong to the mint family, but another

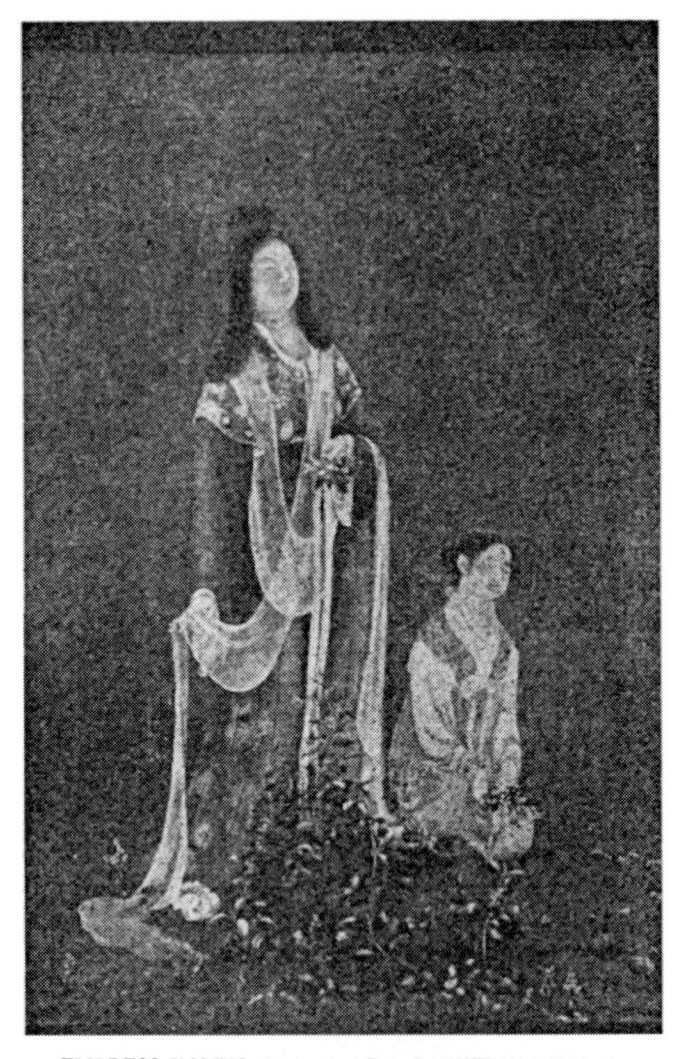

EMPRESS KOMYO (710-793 A.D.) GATHERING HERBS
FOR THE SICK

*Courtesy of Yenching Institute, N. Y., and Publication
Committee, Herb Society of America*

herb called *wood betony* is *Pedicularis canadensis*, with reddish-yellow flowers and fernlike leaves. This herb, belonging to the figwort family, was a simple, well known to the early settlers of America.

BUGLE, *Ajuga reptans*

CALAMINT, *Calamintha officinalis*

CARAWAY, *Carum carvi*

CATNIP, *Nepeta cataria*

*CENTORY, *Centaurea nigra*

CHAMOMILE, *Anthemis nobilis, Matricaria chamomilla*—Both might have been in mediæval gardens.

CHICORY, *Cichorium intybus* (ragged sailors)—The beauty of this herb is not appreciated until given good soil in a garden background.

CLARY, *Salvia sclarea*

COLCHICUM or MEADOW SAFFRON, *Colchicum autumnale*—The action of the drug "colchicine" upon the living cell is of great scientific interest today.

COMFREY, *Symphytum officinale*

CORIANDER, *Coriandrum sativum*

COSTMARY, *Chrysanthemum majus*—This may be the camphor costmary which blooms early with white-rayed flowers, or it may be *C. majus tenacetoides*, which has yellow rayless, tansylike heads.

COWSLIP, *Primula veris*—Medicinally this herb was used in cases of paralysis, which gave it its old name "paralytica."

CRESSES—Introduced by the Romans into Britain.

CUMIN, *Cuminum cyminum*—A Bible herb (Isaiah and Matthew). Its seeds made a most important spice in mediæval times.

DILL, *Anethum graveolens*

DITTANY—This is the common name given to several herbs. *Dictamnus albus* (rue family), the strong-smelling *Fraxinella* of English gardens. *Origanum dictamnus* (mint family), dittany of Crete is its common name; this herb

---

*Probably *Centaurium umbellatum* (centaury) or *Erythraea centaurium* (syn.). Important mediæval simple.

is immortalized by Virgil. Maryland dittany, *Cunila origanoides* (mint family) is a wild herb used as an aromatic tea and found in the south-central states.*

ELECAMPANE, *Inula helenium*—An herb of great medicinal value in the Middle Ages. A tall, rough-leaved yarb with untidy yellow flowers. There are modern horticultural varieties which are really ornamental.

FENNEL, *Foeniculum vulgare*

FEVERFEW, *Matricaria parthenium*—This old "fever herb" is recorded in the Charlemagne Capitulaire, 812 A.D.

FOXGLOVE, *Digitalis purpurea*—A biennial herb with spotted purple flowers. A cardiac stimulant, "digitalis," is extracted from the poisonous leaves of this herb.

GERMANDER, *Teucrium chamaedrys*

GILLY-FLOWERS, or CLOVE PINK, *Dianthus caryophyllus*

HERB ROBERT, *Geranium robertianum*—This fragile wild flower of rocky woodlands was a valuable herb with styptic qualities.

HOLLYHOCK, *Althaea rosea*—The gelatinous roots of *Althea officinalis* are still used commercially.

HONEYSUCKLE, *Lonicera periclymenum*—The "woodbine" of early English poetry was really this honeysuckle (not Ampelopsis).

HOREHOUND, *Marrubium vulgare*

HYSSOP, *Hyssopus officinalis*—The plant mentioned in the Bible was not this herb. The Bible hyssop may have been one of the marjorams.

IRIS—*Iris florentina*, *Iris pallida* and *Iris pseudacorus* are probably the herbs referred to in mediæval lists as "gladiola." From the dried and powdered roots of the first two species the fragrant orris powder of commerce is made.

LAVENDER, *Lavandula officinalis*

LILY, *Lilium candidum*—Although there were several other species used medicinally, the Madonna lily is the herb best known.

---

*See "American Dittany," *The Herbarist*, Publication of the Herb Society of America, 1937.

MARIGOLD, *Calendula officinalis*—Its flowers are still used in cooking. They also make a healing salve.

MUGWORT—Many species were used.

MULLEIN, *Verbascum thapsus*—Its tall stalks of yellow flowers, rising from the broad woolly leaves, have long since given it many significant old-country names—torches, blanket herb.

OXLIP, *Primula elatior*—Teas, vinegars and confections were made from its flowers.

PEONY, *Paeonia officinalis*

PERIWINKLE, *Vinca minor;* also *Vinca major*—This trailing evergreen, with blue or white flowers, was called joy-of-the-ground. Perhaps it was because this herb grew so easily in the shaded, walled enclosures of castle-fortress or monastery it was considered to have much virtue both medicinal and magical.

POPPY, *Papaver somniferum*—This is the tall, pale-flowered poppy, from the capsule of which is extracted opium gum.

PRIMROSE, *Primula vulgaris*—The primrose so loved by the English poets. Also from its flowers was made the famous primrose wine.

ROSE—See "Old Roses," page 57.

ROSEMARY, *Rosmarinus officinalis*

RUE, *Ruta graveolens*

SAFFRON CROCUS, *Crocus sativus*

SPEEDWELL, *Veronica officinalis*—A blue-flowered herb.

SWEETBRIAR, *Rosa eglanteria*

SWEET CICELY, *Myrrhis odorata*

SWEET WOODRUFF, *Asperula odorata*—Recorded about the year 1200.

THYME—Many varieties.

VALERIAN, *Valeriana officinalis*—Garden heliotrope. Red valerian is *Cetranthus ruber;* Greek valerian is *Polemonium caeruleum*.

VERVAIN, *Verbena officinalis*—Common name "herb o' grace." Why this pale-flowered, weedy herb ever became so imbued with magical virtue is a mystery. The Druids revered it. Perhaps the styptic tannic principle found in its stems and leaves bears out the legend, cited by Mrs. Grieves in her Herbal, that the herb was found on the Mount of Calvary and used to staunch the wounds of the Saviour. At any rate, as a very sacred and old-world herb, tuck it away in some corner of your mediæval garden, the only place where it belongs.

VIOLET, *Viola odorata*

VIPER'S BUGLOSS, *Echium vulgare*—A bristly medicinal herb, blue-flowered.

WATERLILY, *Nymphaea odorata*

VALLEY LILY, *Convallaria majalis*—A medicinal herb.

WILD WOAD, *Isatis tinctoria*—The fermented leaves make the famous blue-green dye which Caesar records. Its tall stems of yellow flowers are most decorative in any garden.

WOAD WAXEN, *Genista tinctoria*—This is the "broom" so well known on sandy hillsides, where it began its existence as an escape from Puritan gardens.

YARROW, *Achillea millefolium*—A famous herb of healing.

GARDEN OF POT HERBS

"God who maketh the grass for the cattle and the green herb for the service of man."

There seems to be no one historic background on which to model the modern kitchen garden of pot herbs. For uncounted centuries these plants have been grown with other herbs in all manner of ways for the sustenance and delectation of mankind.

French gardens show the pot herbs delightfully combined with vegetables, and from this influence, perhaps, the hand-cultivated American kitchen garden will become more pleasingly ornamental and attractive.

The condiment herbs, including thyme, marjoram, savory and sage may be planted with the vegetables. Chives, parsley and smallage make trim edgings. Rows of leeks, or other alliums, with their graceful, lilaceous leaves and flowers, offset the fernlike foliage of skirrets and carrots. Purple cabbage in rows between chicory and kale's wrinkled leaves pleases the

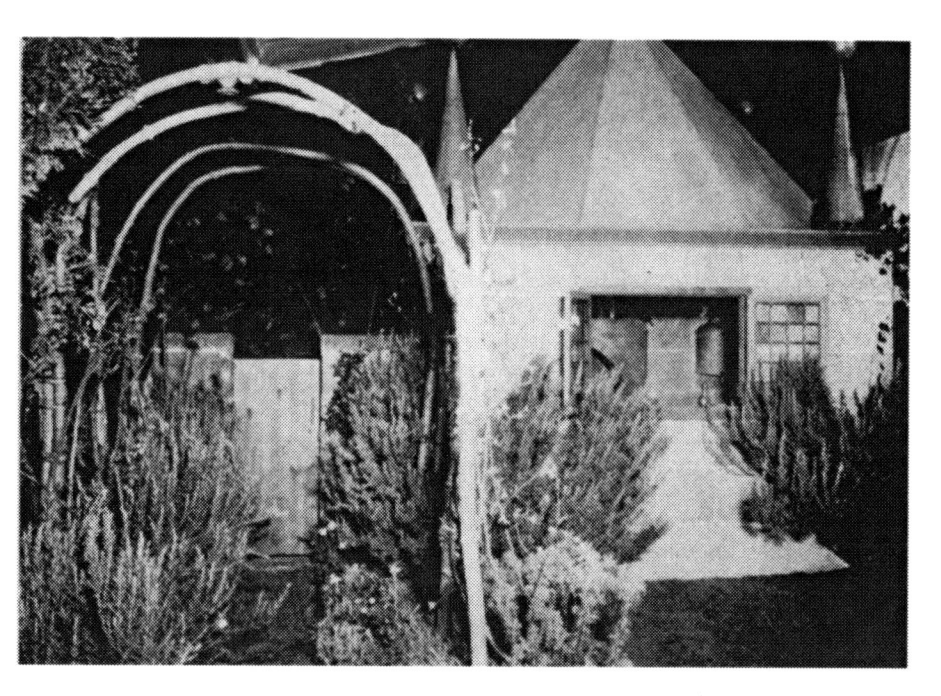

17TH CENTURY STILL HOUSE
Massachusetts Society Flower Show 1935.

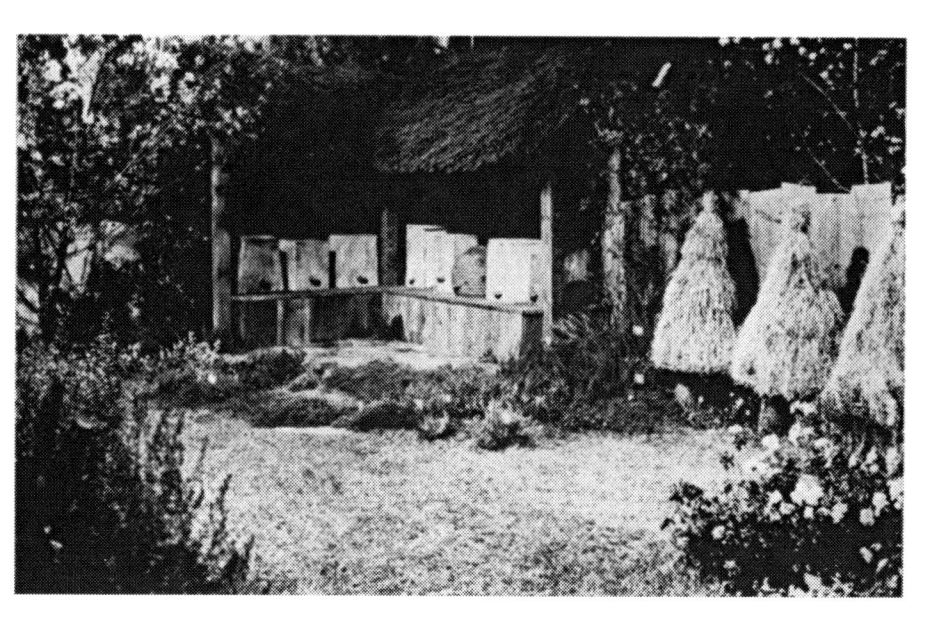

BEE GARDEN, 17TH CENTURY
Massachusetts Horticultural Society Flower Show, 1937.

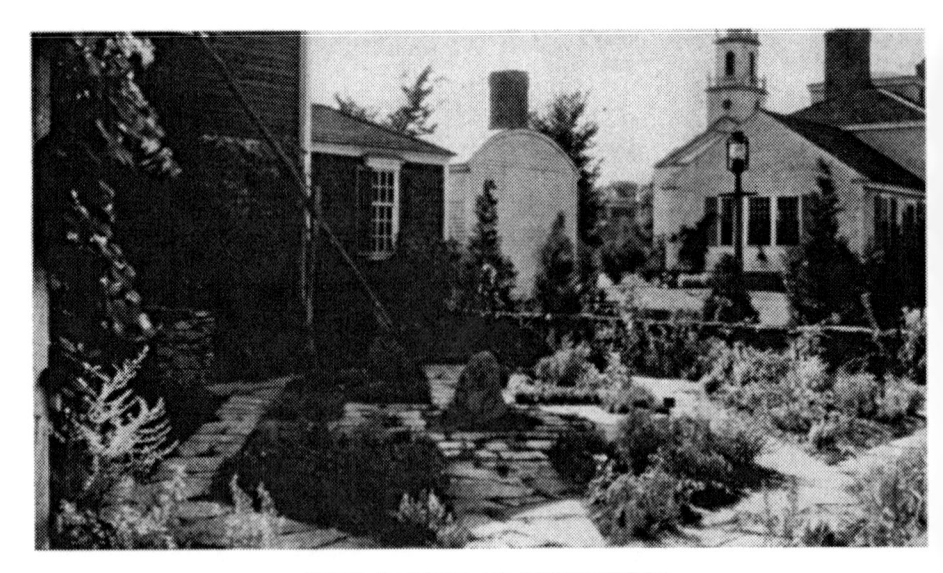

HERB GARDEN AT STORROWTON
West Springfield, Massachusetts

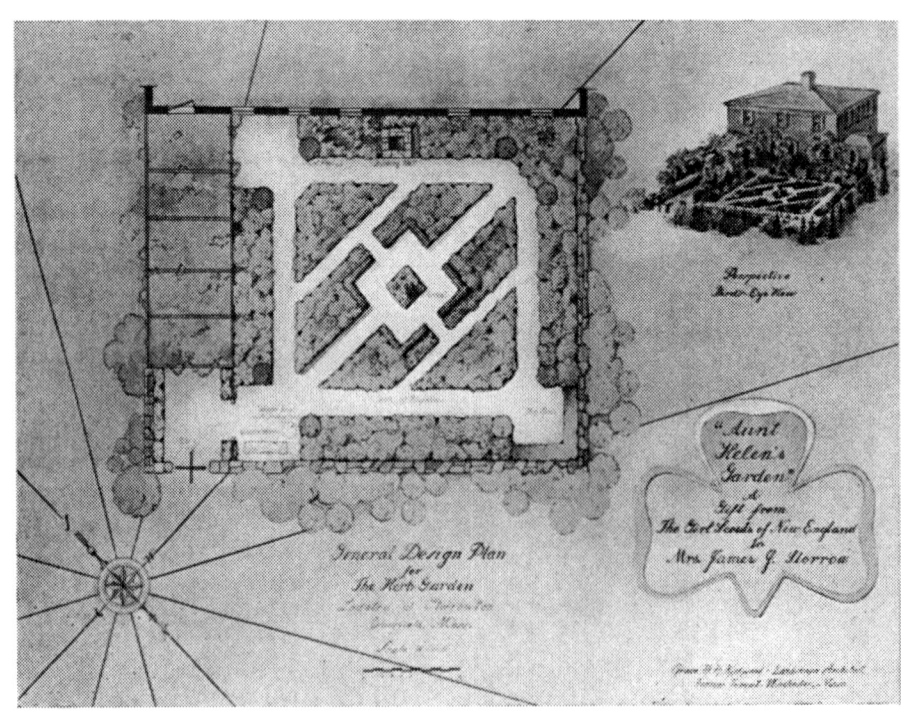

GENERAL DESIGN PLAN FOR THE STORROWTON HERB GARDEN
*Director, Mrs. Charles Newell, West Springfield, Massachusetts.
Designed by Mrs. Samuel Kirkwood.*

eye as part of the whole color scheme. Red and green orach grow where common vegetables need with them a note of color.

The restoration within the last few years of George Washington's kitchen garden at Mt. Vernon has helped educationally to create interest in this kind of gardening.

Very early plant lists include many herbs "for the pot" which, notwithstanding their quaint old names, are just the ancestors of our "improved varieties" of vegetables. (See Mediæval Plant List, page 27.) Smallage is wild celery, and if we allow "Boston Market" to run wild without blanching we shall get, in its green leaves, the richness of flavor that belongs to smallage.

Alexanders are sometimes called "wild lovage." They grow and taste much like celery and, like that herb, must be blanched to be delicate in a salad.

A twelfth-century list of herbs that grew in the garden of an English monastery was compiled by the Abbot, Alexander Neckham. He was a scholarly monk, and himself not much of a gardener, but brought up from childhood in the abbey with Richard the First, he must have absorbed much garden knowledge from the wise horticulturist monks who were his teachers. This list with that of Charlemagne of the ninth century gives us an idea of what pot herbs were eaten in early England and France.

Lettuce was grown in several varieties, as well as all our familiar vegetables. Lady Northcote, in her "Book of Herbs," deplores these prosaic days which have robbed Endive of its virtues. "Once upon a time," she said, "Endive could break all bonds and render the wearer invisible. All its legends are of romantic character and *we* regard it just as a salad herb."

Orachs or arrachs are tall annuals with succulent leaves. One variety is blood red throughout the plant and the type species is bright yellow-green. They are good succulents with which to vary the inevitable spinach.

There are two garden species of sorrel besides the sour-leaved herb of the fields. *Rumex scutatus,* French sorrel, is best for sorrel soup and for salad. Its broad, juicy leaves appear very early in the spring and as we cut them new ones keep appearing until winter. Good King Henry, *Chenopodium Bonus Henricus,* is an herb which looks something like sorrel, a leafy little plant with no particular interest except its name and legends in Teutonic mythology.

Strawberry blite, or blitum as it is called, is a good pot herb as well as ornamental. It has clusters of fleshy, bright red flowers. In places it has escaped from the old gardens.

Skirrets have all but disappeared from nursery lists, but now the modern kitchen garden would be incomplete without their delicately flavored, clustered roots. The Emperor Tiberius liked their anise sweetness so well that he ordered the herb brought for him from Germany. Skirrets came into American gardens before 1770, and many are the early recipes in old cook books for their use, as in skirret pie and in cold salads. Like all the other pot herbs, they need good rich garden soil, loose and not over acid.

Several herbs go by the name of rocket, but this pot herb should not be confused with hesperis, sweet rocket, the night-fragrant biennial of old-fashioned gardens. Rocket, or roquette, genus *Eruca,* is a bitter, rough-leaved plant, sometimes offered in today's market. To be at all palatable, it must be eaten in very young leaf. Another "rocket" is the little hedge mustard which smells of garlic and is an unendurable pest in the garden. In 1599, Gerarde wrote, "Who taketh the seed of Rocket before he be whipped shall be so hardened that he shall easily endure the pain."

Numerous species of the mustard family have been used by man for ages as pot and salad herbs, and a few have survived or have been reinstated in this vitamin-conscious age. As wild herbs they have furnished the pot of rich and poor alike, but in America, whatever their worth may be, they are weeds too rampant to be called wholly epicurean. No exception is St. Barbara's herb, with its showy yellow flowers and shining lyre-shaped leaves. Sometimes it is called wintercress, or yellow rocket. It is so good and piquant in the spring salad that we invite it into the herb garden and think of it as just one of those herbs which "shows by its abundance its good to man."

Cresses, both the horticultural varieties and the water cress of our brooks, are rich in iron as is attested by the reddish color in the leaves of the latter. A soup of water cress is an old headache cure, and Culpepper caustically remarked, "Those who will live in health may use it if they please. If they will not, I cannot help it."

Today we are hearing much of rampion, samphire and rocambole, all pot herbs, tried and true.

Now should every salad lover read John Evelyn's discourse upon salads. In 1699, he wrote his book upon them and called it "Acetaria".*

Rampion (*Campanula rapunculus*) Evelyn calls the "Esculent Campanula" and tells us that the roots have better flavor than radishes. This pot herb, long known in the Old World, came into American gardens about 1800. The stems of lovely light blue bells are ornamental, and this herb does not spread so wildly as the next species very like it, called the "creeping bell-flower" *C. rapunculoides.* Both leaves and roots were eaten raw in salads, or boiled.

Rocambole is an allium, one of the onion tribe, something like garlic but of milder flavor. In 1800, it is listed as one of the American garden esculents. Evelyn remarks that it is "much fitter for ladies' palates than the less gentle garlic." Another allium is moly, yellow garlic, of more interest because it kept Ulysses, who profferred it to Circe, from being changed to a pig.

The shallot is grown for the delicate onion flavor of its "cloves" as the divisions of its bulb are called.

Leeks are associated with early Welsh history and have much graceful beauty.

---

*Happily for us, there is now a faithful reprint of this essay published by the Woman's Committee of the Brooklyn Botanic Garden.

English samphire, *Crithmum maritum* (herbe de St. Pierre), is recorded as growing in American gardens around 1800, when so many esculents were brought in from other countries. In 1936 this plant was shown by Richard Stiles, probably for the first time in America, in an educational exhibit of the Massachusetts Horticultural Society. Few knew the herb other than in those lines of Shakespeare's "King Lear": "Half way down hangs one who gathers samphire, dreadful trade!"

The home of this herb is on English cliffs in rock crevices washed by salty spray. The fleshy, brittle stems and leaves have the same salty, pungent taste as our wild samphire of the New England marshes, and it makes the same good pickle. As to the cultivation of the English samphire, the one plant that I possess was encouraged by a summer mulch of rockweed brought from the seashore.

Renaissance Gardens

In the transition of the herb garden through mediæval, Tudor, Stuart and Victorian periods, the herbs became of less importance. They were never wholly abandoned, but with the discovery of new lands came a period of plant introductions and exchange between countries.

It is said that no lovelier herb gardens ever were than those of the sixteenth-century Tudor mansion, and happily we have beautiful word pictures of them in the immortal verse of the Elizabethan poets, Drayton, Spenser, Herrick and Shakespeare.

Also the fairly peaceful, well-governed years encouraged many garden writers whose early volumes are eagerly sought by collectors today. In their descriptions, plant lists, garden design and wisdom is the background for three centuries of American gardening.

A very early treatise of this period was that of Mayster Jon Gardener, written just before 1450 and called "Feate of Gardening." He records over a hundred plants and trees of which every one has herbal significance. But by his day

EARLY PERIODS AND DESIGNS OF THE HERB GARDEN 37

may we not suspect that roses, lilies, violets, primulas and iris were grown for beauty as well as for medicine?

Also, in this list there is not one species which we may not find today somewhere in American gardens. A few mentioned are ambrosia, betony, borage, bugle, calamint, comfrey, chamomile, cresses, clary, English dittany (fraxinella), garlic, horehound, mints, catnip, parsley, radish, rue, saffron, sage, savory, thyme, fennel, woodruff, hyssop, lavender.

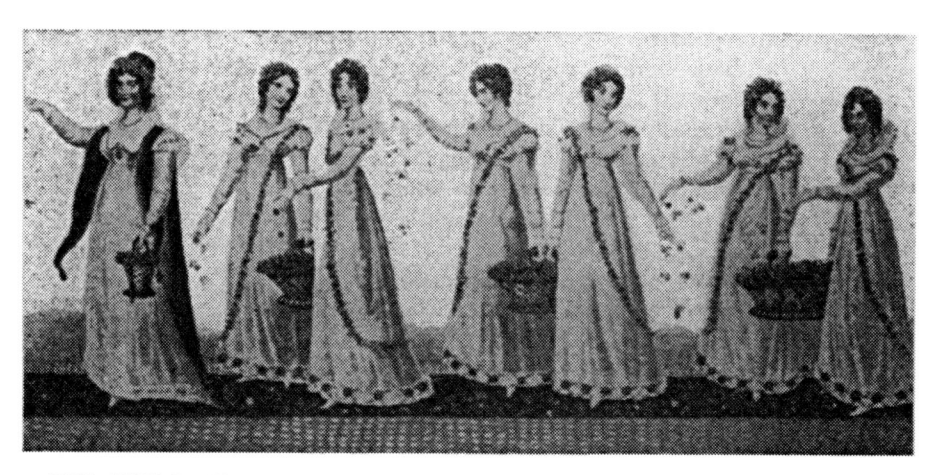

THE KING'S HERB WOMAN, MISS FELLOWES, AND HER MAIDS, 1821*
From Naylor's Coronation of George IV

Herbs we have long thought of as weeds are included in these lists, yarrow, tansy, agrimony, motherwort, pimpernel, buttercup, St. John's-wort, teasle. Besides these were all the pot herbs included in mediæval lists.

Another herbal of which we hear much was "A New Herbal" by one William Turner, 1551.

Even more famous for its sound advice was Thomas Tusser's "One Hundred Points of Good Husbandry for House-

---
*See *The Herbarist*, 1938, Publication Herb Society of America, "The King's Herb-Woman," Elizabeth Wade White.

wives." This was so popular that over twenty editions followed the first.

But of all the old books that the herb gardener of today knows and loves best, are the great English herbals of Gerarde and Parkinson published in 1595 and 1633.

To be sure the vast fund of information contained in these volumes is not wholly from the writers' own observation and research, but much was drawn from the accounts of the great teachers and physicians who had preceded them by centuries.

Both Gerarde and Parkinson were in charge of great gardens which were full of plants from all the known world then explored, and their books are invaluable today for the choice descriptions of gardens and plants of those years, as well as for their wise herbal therapy.

Through modern reprints, many of these books are available to the American gardener, and he who chooses to make a Renaissance garden today needs only planting space and access to the alluring writings of that period.

Another garden on which to build is described by Francis Bacon in his essay "Of Gardens," 1625. Whether this garden be real or an ideal of his dreams, its beauty is unsurpassed, and we read and reread "God Almightie first Planted a Garden. And indeed it is the Purest of Humane Pleasures." No feature of the Renaissance garden is omitted in this essay. Fragrance and soft colors are treated as of paramount importance.

Walks were turfed and planted with sweet herbs that "crushed and trodden do perfume the aire most delightfully." Therefore Bacon bids us "set whole alleys of them to have pleasure when you walk or tread." The alleys were "pleached" by weaving the over-arching branches of parallel rows of trees, making a long, covered passage "by which you may goe in shade into the garden," and "that when the wind blowes sharpe you may walke as in a gallery."

Tudor gardeners used hawthorn, elm, hornbeam for "pleaching," and American gardeners frequently make use of

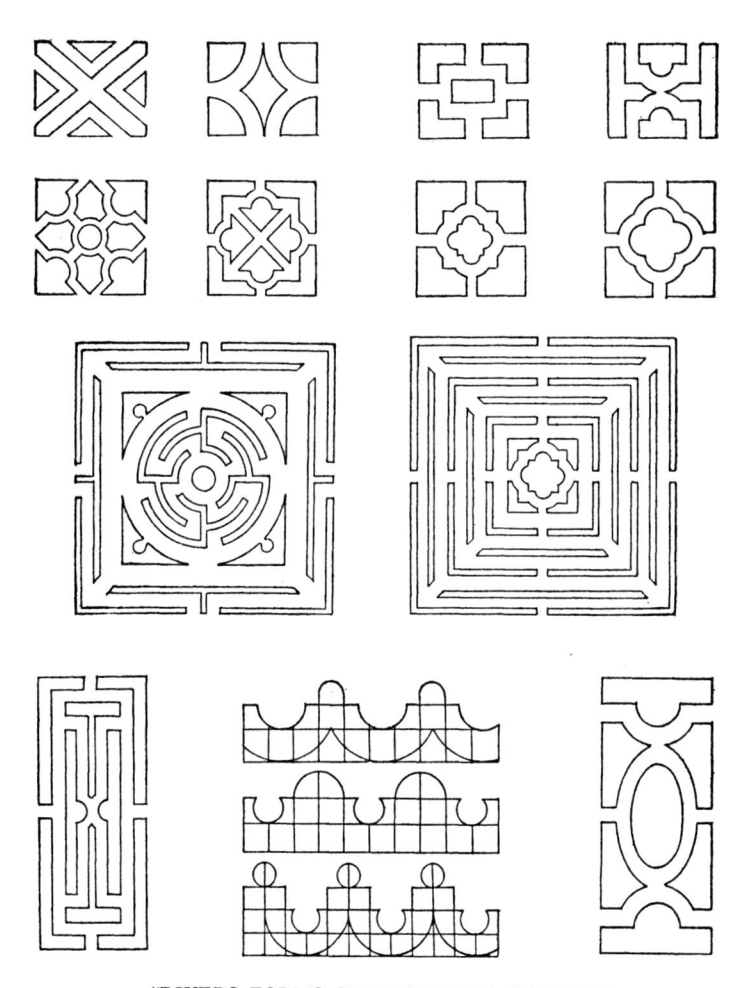

"DIVERS FORMS OR PLOTS FOR GARDENS"

Now that the herb garden has again come into its own it may be interesting to consider some of the designs used in the early 18th century as a possible motif for our present-day gardens. "The Complete English Gardner," written in 1704 by Leonard Meager, presents "Divers forms or plots for gardens," a few of which are shown here.
—Frances T. Norton

arbor vitae. In "Much Ado About Nothing," Shakespeare suggests the tunnel made by these overarching branches: "A pleached bower where honeysuckles ripened by the sun, forbid the sun to enter."

Hedges of this period were built for "use and delight." Hawthorn got its name "quick-set" from its popularity as a quick-growing hedge tree.

Privet, yew, eglantine, firethorn (*Pyracantha*) and cornel are spoken of as for "good impenetrable hedges."

Lord Bacon advises that the hedge be "raised upon a Banke, not steep, but gently sloped of some Six Foot all set with flowers of sweet smell."

Summer houses or "herbers" were covered and enclosed with the sweetest of fragrant vines, which were called "arch herbs."

Fountains of varied and beautiful workmanship seem always to be an important part of Tudor gardens.

Equally ornate are the table and carved seats around which knights and their ladies gathered.

We read of heraldic animals of all kinds carved of wood, and surmounting pillars. Bacon speaks disparagingly of artificial appurtenances so common in the great gardens of this time, and does not like "Images cut out of Juniper or other Garden stuff." "Topiary work is for children," he thinks. But the practice of cutting privet, yew and even rosemary into warriors, lions rampant and animals was then common in the gardens of the rich.

In his essay, Bacon has much to tell of the "Mount of some Pretty Height, leaving the wall of the Enclosure Brest high, to look abroad into the fields."

We read of raised beds for the herbs. They were boarded with slabs of wood much as we may see them today when we try to keep roots from spreading.

Garden writings around 1600 speak of the maze, but its making seems to have been a pretty pastime long after Stuart days.

If the paths are intricate in their inlocking and their enclosing hedge walls high and thick, in a small guarding tower, raised high above all, is posted a sentinel to guide the wanderers back to the starting point.

In the Stuart gardens, the maze was just a garden plaything made with low shrubs outlining the winding paths. Southernwood, rosemary, lavender, rue, marjorams and basils were used. How sweet a game to play in that leisurely age, when, brushed by the gowns of the ladies, the herbs gave out their fragrance.

Didymus Mountain wrote his book "The Gardener's Labyrinth" in 1577 and it is suggested that this might have been the textbook from which Shakespeare made his own knot garden at Stratford.

Laid out in intricate patterns are the "knot gardens" which became famous in the days of the Renaissance and about which we may read in many books. These are gardens of bewildering design and motive, the beds edged with rue, hyssop, box and santolina, thrift and thyme. Perhaps they are heart-shaped beds, lavender-filled, entwined by serpentine coils of forget-me-nots and marigolds.

Any gardener with a liking for geometric circles, curves and angles or straight lines may build himself a "knot" provided he places it pleasantly in appropriate architectural setting with Tudor hedges and other appurtenances. Old gardening books of this age picture most intriguing patterns.

If watches and clocks were not now so common we should still be measuring time by the movement of the shadow cast on the garden sundial, and in any period reproduction, the garden is really more interesting with this ancient timekeeper, which was well known in gardens of Tudor and Stuart times.

The circles of the Astrolabe were used by the Greeks in observing the stars and position of the heavenly bodies, and this classic instrument is today a choice find for the garden. That it did appear in the very early herb gardens of England is surmised, and by its dictation, that none of their healing efficacy be lost, was governed the culling of herbs. Sweet basil was governed by Mars in the Scorpion, and betony, for which many a man "would sell his coat" was Jupiter's herb in Aries. Burnet, a precious herb, little inferior to betony, was gathered under the sun's auspices alone. An inventive lover of herbs and their symbolism paints on her garden labels that astronomical sign of the planet which governs each little medicinal plant.

The bee skep rightly appears in any garden at any time, and there is no more useful or decorative feature.

Shakespeare gardens made with more or less accuracy have been popular ever since the restoration of the Stratford garden. As to the actual herbs, shrubs and trees that grew in his garden, we rely upon the poet's reference to them in his plays and the plant lists of the times.

Gerarde's London garden was not far from Shakespeare's home, and he must have known it and its herbs well.

A Shakespeare garden should have in it, we know, all those old-fashioned, lowly fragrants of the day, and no modern "improved variety" wedged in for its gayer colors and greater size.

So replete with romance, poetry and sentiment are the gardens of all the Renaissance years, that we cannot grow their herbs without sensing that never-aging verse of the Elizabethan poets.

*Partial List of Herbs for a Shakespeare Garden**

(The Botanical species, if given in other lists, is not repeated here.)

Aconite
Angelica
Balm
Box, dwarf tree and gilded
    varieties

Carnations
Chamomile
Chaste tree, *Vitex agnus-castus*
Chaucer daisy, *Bellis*

---

*See *The Herbarist*, 1936, Publication Herb Society of America, "Shakespeare's Flowers," Elizabeth Wade White.

Cowslips
Crow-flowers, which might have been ragged robin, *Lychmis floscuculi* or *Scilla nonscripta*
Crown imperial
Cuckoo buds or buttercups
Cuckoo flowers, mustards
Daffodil or crow-bell
Dian's bud, *Artemisia*
Dill
Eglantine or sweetbriar
Fennel
Ferns
Foxgloves
Harebells
Heartsease
Honeysuckle
Hyssop
Ivy
Lady-smock, *Cardamine pratensis*
Larkspur
Lavender
Lilies
Long-purples, which might have been an orchis
Marjoram
Mint
Mulberry tree
Old roses
Onions
Oxlips
Pansies
Parsley
Peony
Pinks
Poppy
Primroses or hose in hose (double primrose)
Rue
Samphire
Savory
Snapdragon
Southernwood
Striped or streaked gillyflower
Stocks
Sweet Williams
Thistle
Thymes
Violets
Winking Mary bud or marigold, *Calendula officinalis*
Wormwood

Now comes the period in herb gardening when the famous Stuart gardens of England begin to link us with our own Colonial gardens. It was the period of interesting plant exchange between the mother country and her colonies. "African" marigolds from Mexico, four o'clocks from South America, sunflowers and goldenrods from the northern continent traveled into the English gardens. As their gardeners pushed farther and farther into the background the humble, fragrant simples to make room for the gay novelties, "outlandish plants," the herbalist mourned the lost prestige of his herbs.

But just as eagerly did the American colonists receive into their gardens, north and south, the precious simples of the homeland.

Frequent and amusing references are found in that early correspondence. In a letter of William Logan to Sir Thomas Bincks, published in the Pennsylvania section of "Gardens of Colony and State," he ordered sent to him from England "Catipelars and Snales." Parkinson describes them in his "Paradisus." I have grown the funny little things in my own garden from seed. And I do not wonder that the Colonial women wanted them again as "surprises in salad and soups."

It is consoling to think that in connection with the seventeenth-century Still-Room* of England the herb garden remained of paramount importance. The Still-Room garden was small and tended by the housewife herself and her maids. From its worts were made electuaries, which were the soothing herb-and-honey medicinals; robs, the hot drinks; salves, sweet washing waters, perfumes and other "conceits."

Although the Still-Room was never the kitchen of the palace or mansion wherein the meals were prepared, yet it was a vitally necessary room where were collected the products of the herb garden, and medicinals were distilled. In the famous Still-Room books all manner of choice recipes were collected.

The apothecary physicians of England and Europe were greatly interested in American herbs of healing and the herbal therapy of the American Indian.

Tobacco was a medicinal narcotic and used in surgery before it became a "smoke." Quinine, witch hazel, lobelia and many more herbs were introduced into the great London physic garden at Chelsea.

In Stuart times the kitchen gardens were so well supplied

---

*See *The Herbarist*, 1935, Publication Herb Society of America, "The 17th Century Still-Room," Adeline P. Cole.

with numerous varieties of vegetables and pot herbs that America had less to offer that was new. But the white potato and Jerusalem artichoke grew slowly, from the year 1585, to extreme popularity.

After all it is for our own loved and unpretentious herb gardens of America, old and new, that this book is compiled. If I have lingered too long over old-world gardens it is because they and their stories are the chief source of all that we know today of the oldest kind of gardening and the ancient herbs.

With this background, aside from the herbal therapy of the American Indian, little has been added to our knowledge of herb lore and usage in three American centuries.

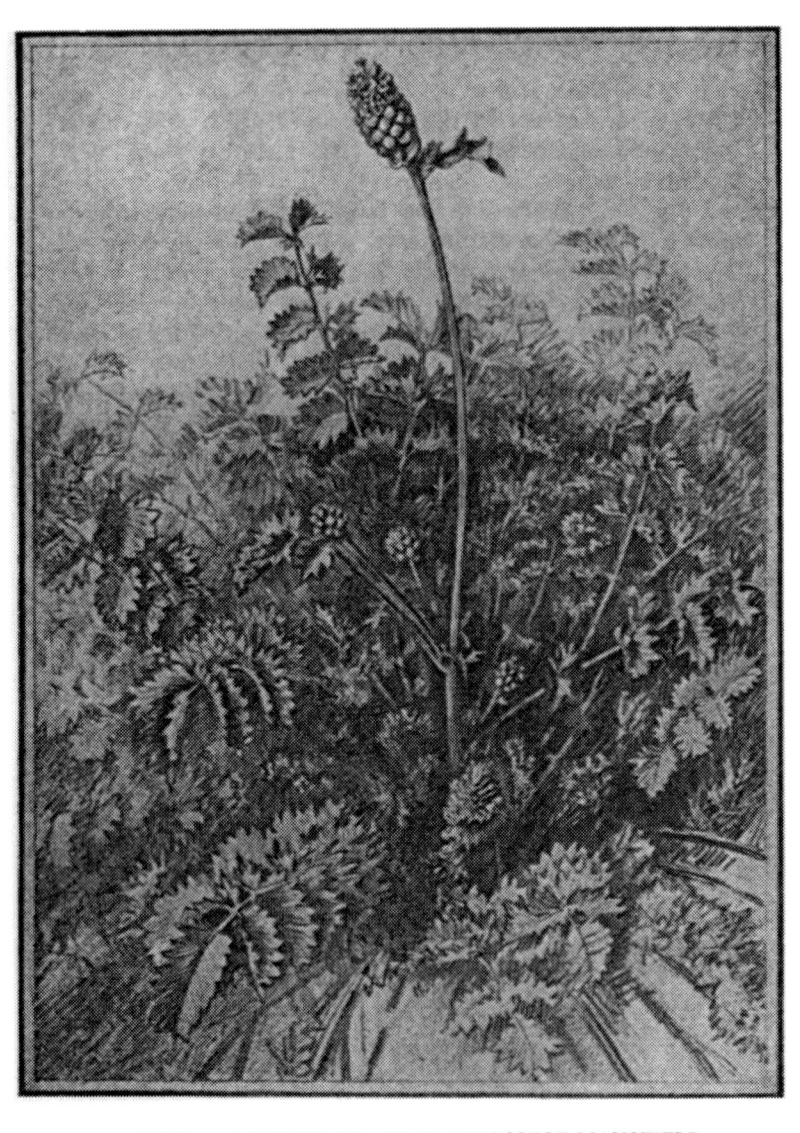

BURNET — A PENCIL DRAWING BY LOUISE MANSFIELD

Owned by the Herb Society of America
One of plates included in "An Artist's Herbal" (*Macmillan,* 1937)

CHAPTER II

COLONIAL GARDENS

JOHN JOSSELYN, Gentleman, about fifty years after the landing of the Pilgrims wrote a book about plants in New England gardens. The now common weeds, plantain, nettle, sow thistle, shepherd's purse, chickweed, knot grass, couch grass, dandelion and mullein were not known before this time in North America. These weeds came to New England perhaps with their own herbal history of past usefulness to man, or perhaps by chance.

The recorded list of commonly-cultivated pot herbs and simples is here repeated for the convenience of the reader who may not have access to "New England Rarities Discovered": "Cabbage, Lettuce, Parsley, Marygold (Calendula), French Mallow, Chervil, Burnet, Winter and Summer Savory, Time (Thyme), Sage, Carrots, Red Beetes, Radishes, Purslain (Pusley), Pease of all sorts, Spearmint, Featherfew (Feverfew) prospereth exceedingly, and Botrys (Ambrosia) not at all. Southernwood is no plant for this country, nor is Rosemary. White Satten (Honesty) groweth pretty well."

From the Massachusetts Bay Colony, as the settlers pioneered farther into the new wildernesses, north and west, the garden herbs spread, sharing their vicissitudes and fortunes of migration.

In Plymouth, by the Pilgrim Spring, grows today the descendant of a mint, planted, if not in the first year of the settlement, then very soon after. Alice Morse Earle, in "Old Time Gardens," makes live again for us the devotion and sacrifice which attended that mint during its sea voyage to start with the Pilgrims its own kind in the new world.

I discovered ambrosia, or Jerusalem oak, and the golden apple mint on the Kennebec River growing near the last of the old tide mills. "How long had it been there?" I inquired. "It had never *not* grown there," was the answer. I feel that in the old town records of Arrowsic might be found the date of its honorable establishment with the first settlers.

West over the Alleghenies, early in the last century, "Johnny Appleseed" carried, with his seedling apple trees and religion, the lore of garden herbs to the frontier families of Ohio and Indiana. So significant is one stanza in "When Johnny Appleseed Comes," found in Elisabeth Peck's recent volume of verse, that I have begged permission to print it here. Says "Granny" to Johnny:

"Might you have any catnip seed?
The hogs used my nice bed for their feed.
Your horehound grows like some common weed, Appleseed
Johnny,
And the pennyroyal patch is a sight to see.
How shall I make that dog-fennel tea,
When chills and fever lay hold of me?
And have you any catnip, Appleseed Johnny?"

"Plant the seed by a wet moon, Granny."

It is obvious to even the most skeptical, therefore, that any garden reproduction or restoration of Colonial period must depend upon the local backgrund of tradition and history.

"Gardens of Colony and State," published by the Garden Club of America, is replete with illustrations of gardens, existing and bygone, old garden correspondence and plant lists with clues to their introduction into American gardens.

Every herb gardener finds delight in making the project garden of his dreams, and some have come true. A friend described to me enthusiastically her "Wheel of Thyme" in a sunny New Hampshire homestead. Between the spokes of an old cartwheel are planted the different varieties of thyme, that herb so symbolizing the past industry of the ancient wagon wheel. I hope that wheel is rimmed with quaint ger-

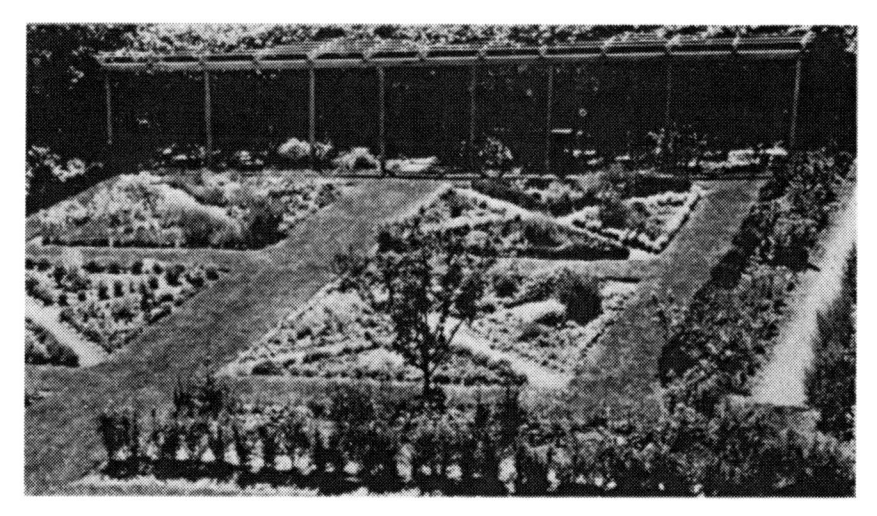

FORMAL HERB GARDEN OF PARDEE MORRIS HOUSE 1685-1779
This garden, designed by Mrs. Thomas E. Hayward, is at Morris Cove, Connecticut.

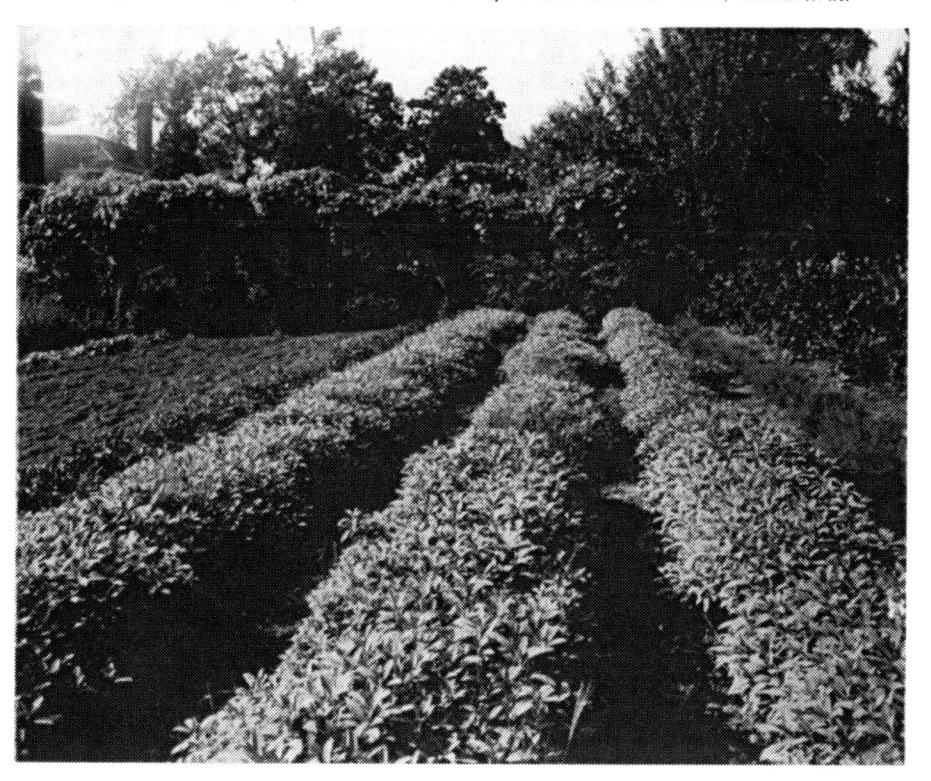

EXPERIMENTAL PLOT OF SAGE — VARIETY "HOLT'S MAMMOTH"
Brookby Farm, Wenham, Mass. "Cuttings" were set 1930 and plants have been cropped for drying twice each year 1931-1938.

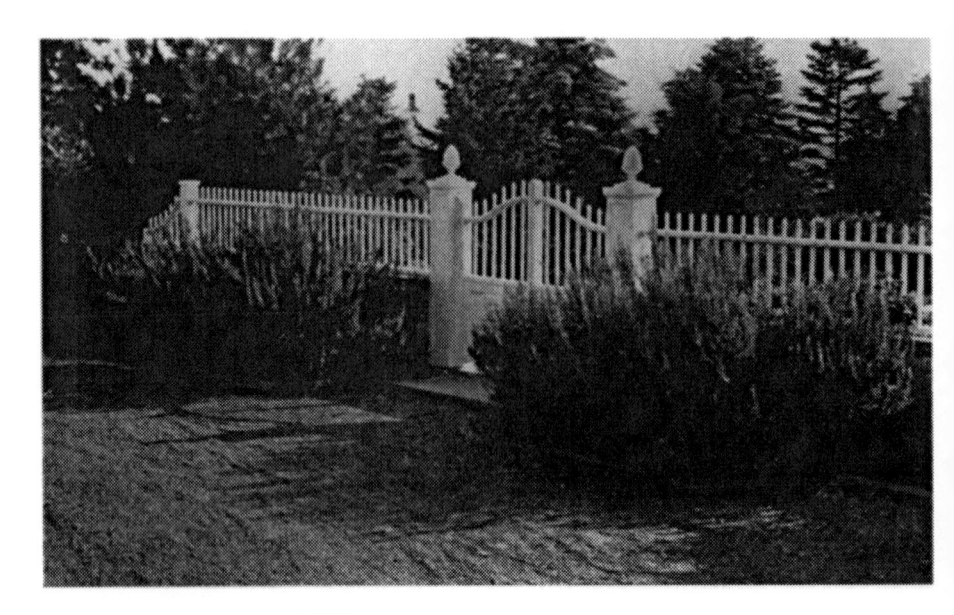

ROSEMARY AT AN ENTRANCE GATE
Home of Mr. and Mrs. Geoffrey Whitney, Woods Hole, Massachusetts.

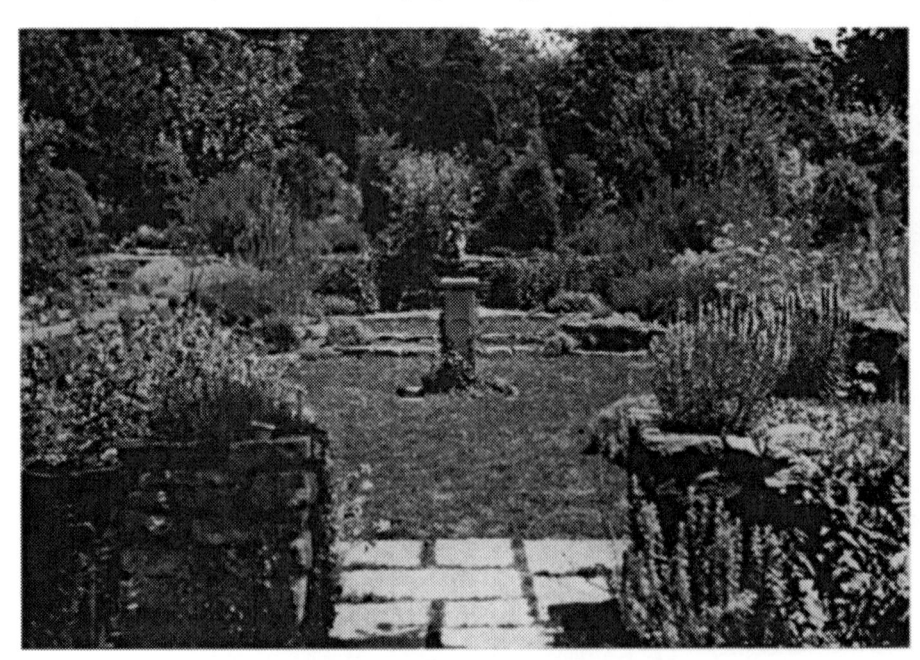

WALLED HERB GARDEN
Home of Mr. and Mrs. Geoffrey Whitney, Woods Hole, Massachusetts.
A wonderfully beautiful planting which shows the adaptability of herbs in these surroundings.

mander, for Gerard says "Its flowers be of a gallant blew colour, made of four small leaves apiece, standing orderly on the tops of the tender spriggy spraies"! And according to his observations germander "do love to grow in rough and rocky grounds such as be open to the aire and sun, and in gardens they do easily prosper." It may be that the hub is of chamomile white and gold, signifying patience in a changing world. The spokes themselves are outlined in silver thyme between the green and gray leaves of the other varieties.

The ladder herb garden was new to me, but an "old" idea. It was made close by a friendly mansion on the Hudson in New York, and seemed to just "belong" in this setting.

The different herbs are grown between the rungs of two ladders set parallel in the ground. A long path between the ladders is broken in the center with a wheel of thymes. At the end of this path is a wooden bench where, between fragrant bushes of roses and tall herbs, one may sit and find enjoyment and peace in contemplation of the whole. The garden is enclosed in a white picket fence and is entered by a gate which faces the seat, and is flanked by tall bushes of artemisias.

The smallest herb garden that I know in this country is a lovable little affair built within four walls. This garden has been successfully reproduced from one which might have belonged to the fair lady of some Norman castle. The enclosed borders grow many kinds of herbs. A dovecote is in the corner as should be, and, true to tradition, the white fantail invariably appears when the garden door opens. Narrow turret stairs lead to a view of wide fields and dunes.

The Colonial herb garden is perhaps the most often tried experiment today and is the correct adjunct for the Cape Cod cottage type of house, picket fenced or hedged with box or privet. Here all kinds of "lovesome" flowers for "posies" and domestic uses find their way — sweet herbs, lemon verbena, sweet geraniums, mallows, dittany and what not.

There is a modern adaptation of the English Queen Anne architecture of 1700 now being used for small suburban developments. The jutting angles of these little homes open up so many sunny nooks for landscape gardening befitting this period, that it is a real pity for the house owner not to avail himself of his opportunity to evolve a period garden of sweet and other herbs. Though it be small, it will still have room for many sweet-scented herbs with spring flowers of crocus, hyacinth, snow drop and fritillaries in the shelter of box hedging and saffron crocus in September. All flowering herbs, safflower around the blue-green hyssop, hollyhocks, Canterbury bells and foxgloves, rejoice in the friendly proximity of the brick walls of the house. The walks are turfed and outlined with staggered bricks, between which thymes, marjorams and winter savory fall in clouds of sweetness.

It takes courage and true reverence for the past to create a real "yarb patch" which shall as far as we know be in keeping with the perfect type of the early seventeenth-century farmhouse of New England.

A garden in the historic old Deacon Goodale farm in Marlborough, Massachusetts, shows how the yarbs might have been grown in the eighteenth century. It also reveals how truly beautiful an old "yarb patch" must have been.

There is no particular design or reason in the planting other than that the herbs are planted in places where they could be easily reached by the housewife for all household purposes. A broad grass path separates the pot herbs and the vegetables from the cooking and medicinal herbs.

Basils, purple and green, great and small chives, parsley, sorrel, carrots, tarragon, parsnip, skirrets, strawberries, spinach, and Good King Henry border one side of the path. In the background are sunflowers and single red and white hollyhocks. The tall mallows were not grown for their flowers alone, but for the soft, gelatinous salve extracted from the "stamped" root. Bouncing Bet is there, for its roots were used to make cleansing, soapy waters.

On the other side of the path is an old pear tree and a dipping well in a sunken tub. Woodruff and forget-me-nots, white violets and chamomile run riot under the tree and out of its bounds. Scented geraniums, lemon verbena, heliotrope, stiff little bushes of thyme, gray and green lavender, rosemary, santolina and mignonette are close to the border for picking and sniffing as we stroll up the path. High in the background stand the tall and stately tiger lilies, angelica and lovage, and against the wall a patch of woolly apple mint. Thick southernwood bushes flank either side of the path's end. There is color the summer through from the hyssops, blue, white and pink; salvias, blue, purple and white; clary, bee balms, and all kinds of mints. The creeping thymes and calamints are everywhere. Tansy, yarrow, and elder bushes are over in one corner. Dill, fennel, caraway, rue, borage, and anchusa, in all their soft shades of foliage-green and flower colors add to the bewildering blending of herb fragrance, which is so unlike that from any other garden.

On both sides of the path are big patches of common sage, that herb of wisdom and immortality, always useful in household economy, which lived ever in complete sympathy with its human family. This whole garden is enclosed by a stone wall backed by a rail fence, and its entrance is through a slab gate between great clumps of the burnet rose.

There are hop vines and honeysuckles and a stone with the zodiac signs of the heavens under whose guidance grew all herbs.

If we would copy the rambling Colonial garden of simples in a modern New England setting, let it be a sunny lot surrounded by tall red cedars and sweetbriar or eglantine, a hedge such as Josselyn describes. On wet spring days, the cedars glisten with orange "may apples," those curious parasitic fungi which by the doctrine of signatures proclaimed their healing value to man. Soon their color is followed by the pink flowers of eglantine, whose long spicy sprays lie on the dark cedar branches and entwine among them. In winter, protected as they are, it is long before the color leaves the red hips.

The outer edge of cedar may be broken occasionally with a shrub of witch hazel and spice bush, for the early settlers in the country transplanted from the woods to their home yards the medicinal shrubs that made "quick hedges" and division lines. Spice bush gives the earliest yellow in spring and witch hazel the last gold of autumn.

The corners should, of course, harbor the drooping snowdrifts of the elder blossoms — for no herb gardens may rightly be without them. "Mother Elder," our forefathers called this shrub. It was the "Guardian of the Herb Garden, and from its shelter, on Midsummer Night's eve, one might see fairies." "Rue kept off the serpents" and "dill was the witches' herb."

There will be a place for all those old-fashioned favorites that grew in our grandmothers' gardens, foxgloves, lupins, larkspurs, Canterbury bells, sweet rocket, and honesty or silver sixpence. The peonies should be in keeping with other flowers of that period, the old, semi-double, red variety. Plant all the old-fashioned roses that you may find in hidden corners of New England, Harrison yellow, and the semi-double fragrant white roses with gold centers which belong with the dignity of old New England villages.

The spring-flowering herbs are as necessary in the New England herb garden as the midsummer lilies. Daffodils, snowdrops, and the winter's aconite are never more lovely than coming up through the green of thymes. In August, saffron bulbs should be planted that we may not miss, the following October, their pale␣croxuslike flowers, from which hang, pendent, the bright yellow stigmas. These with colchicum's rosy clumps usually bring gay color to an end in the herb garden.

No matter where we embed heartsease and ambrosia, with its red-veined leaves, we shall find them next year in every nook and corner of the herb garden, the Johnny-jump-ups with their comical little faces looking at us from the hedgerows.

Gill-over-the-ground is a rampant, spreading herb, but some cold, dark north corner may need just what its trailing stems, beset with shining crenulate leaves and blue flowers, may give us. Hyacinth and yellow "daffys" are enchanting planted in their midst.

The sweet coltsfoot (*Petasites*), is a huge ground cover with enormous leaves and very early, fragrant tufts of flowers before the leaves appear. This is the "winter heliotrope" of English gardens and it may be "just the herb" for some wild, unused corner.

Sweet woodruff is dainty ground cover for partial shade, and likes the same loose, gravelly soil that white bloodroot and yellow coltsfoot enjoy. These last two, however, must be ruthlessly thinned out for the broad leaves, which follow the blooms, cover everything.

An herb garden with all those sweet things, sweet rocket, old-fashioned wall flower, cherry pie (which is heliotrope), lemon verbena, mignonette and sweet geraniums — every variety you can lay your hand upon — is the herb garden of our colonies in the years around 1800. These plants make fragrant and interesting additions in long herb borders, filling in bare spaces left by spring herbs, squills, hyacinth and fritillarias, or the daffodils. Their leaves and blossoms may be used for jellies and posies, and every dried leaf and petal saved for potpourri.

In the formal herb bed of small dimensions it is best to use only those sweet-scented geraniums which are dwarf and compact in their growth, like the citron and nutmeg varieties. The fuzzy-leaved mint geranium and some skeleton-leaved varieties are rather sprawly.

The mints must go in the shady, damp parts of this garden, with their creeping root stalks confined in sunken tubs which are bottomless. Otherwise, the garden may become "all mints."

If this garden is designed with individual herb beds, they must be edged with herbs, low or carefully trimmed. Use parsley, chervil, chives, thrift or clipped hyssop. Box is more hardy in New England than we have been led to believe. Cuttings of *Buxus sempervirens* may be taken in the spring and rooted successfully under shrubbery or in flats of sand. If left undisturbed, and covered with leaves the following winter, after two years the tiny well-rooted plants may be set out to make the beginning of an herb border. If the cuttings are taken from old bushes, long inured to New England winters, they in turn make more resistant plants. The beds may hold any number of combinations for color.

Today a garden picture calls for varied foliage, shade and textures in combination with intense vividness of color. Restfulness is the note sought nowadays in our garden schemes and the herb garden has gentle appeal to all senses. This after all is the purpose of gardens. They must give us rest and peace and just enough stimulation in their fragrance for a harmonious whole.

This is felt when we stand over a bed of scented geraniums, lemon verbenas, heliotrope, and hybrid roses of which so many are beautiful yet scentless.

Fern-leaved chervil combines with sweet marjoram, burnet and the bushy thymes. Cerinthe or the honey herb is attractive with summer savory and borage. The purple sweet basil is lovely with giant hyssop (*Agastache*) and mint bush (*Eschscholtzia*) but this last aromatic bush is a later acquisition.

In our herb garden, we may like to experiment with the less known of the so-called "new varieties" given under the list of sweet-herb genera, but we must remember that nothing ever takes the place of the "old herbs," the particular species used for generations in medicine and cookery.

Through these beds may run formal little paths of turf, brick or flag stone. If of the latter, leave wide strips of earth between them. Here chamomile and the carpeting thymes, white, purple, and pink, take root readily and never resent man's tread upon their fragrance.

But whichever way these paths run, always plan to bring them to the sundial in the center. A circular bed of rich loam around this could be planted with Madonna lilies, larkspur and aconite. Another combination would be the lavender, sweet-scented geraniums and heliotrope. Or low-growing plants of thymes, calamints or evergreen savories may be preferred.

Parkinson, the last of the great herbalists, mourns that

period in the latter part of the sixteenth century when many a "faire flower" was relegated to the "garden of pleasure." Left behind, ignominiously out of sight in the kitchen garden, were their modest companions of bygone centuries, the sweet herbs for healing, cookery and strewing — rue, thyme, marjoram and many others.

For nearly four hundred years the Madonna lily has been a habitant of the "flower garden," its history buried in ancient herbals. Now, for its own sweet sake and for the memories of its great healing and symbolism, let us restore it to its proper place, the garden of herbs. Here, after all, it looks most content, its roots undisturbed and shaded by its friends of old.

> *Opening upon level plots*
> *Of crowned lilies standing near*
> *Purple spiked lavender.*
> — Tennyson's "Ode to Memory."

The story of the rose is the same. Of as ancient a lineage as the lily, it has been loved since the dawn of history for its beauty, fragrance and beneficent healing. Rose petals steeped and boiled with honey made the famous remedy, honey of roses, for sore throats and ulcerated mouths. And to some Devonshire ancestor of our own country people is traced the recipe for that soothing lotion of the early Colonists — rose vinegar. Over a jar of dried rose petals pure vinegar was poured, and there was no greater relief for aching heads than clean linen wrung out in this refreshing liquid.

> *"The rose distills a healing balm,*
> *The beating pulse of pain to calm."*

There are vines, of course, which may properly be included in our herb gardens. The hop is a lovely asset if the vine can be sprayed often enough to keep the hop caterpillar from eating it to bare stems. The foliage is attractive with large leaves which look something like woodbine, and the female flowers hang in festoons of soft green catkins. Dried, these have a soporific fragrance and make wonderful "sleep pillows." Indeed, in country corners of New England this is the best known remedy for neuralgia and toothache. The young shoots are good "greens" in the spring mixture of boiled pot herbs, dandelions, brakes, nettles and lambs-quarters. The Romans ate hops — why not we? But not until the seventeenth century did the flowers of this vine supplant ground ivy, wormwood, yarrow and woodsage in the brewing of ale.

Like the hop vine, the honeysuckle makes a picturesque background for an old herb garden, particularly if that garden is an adjunct of a rambling stone wall. There are about one hundred and fifty kinds of honeysuckle which grow in the cooler portions of the world, but the fragrant flowers of *Lonicera caprifolium*, the Italian honeysuckle, and *L. periclymenum*, the English wild honeysuckle, were probably the most frequently grown for their medicinal lotion.

Before 1700 formal gardening in the Colonial settlements had no place in that determined struggle for permanent homes, but in the peaceful years of the next century, American gardens came into being. Then there revived and developed tremendous interest in horticulture and agricultural pursuits. Under European influences, stately Georgian mansions were built, and around them were made the famous Colonial gardens. These were beautifully landscaped and fitted with a flora rich with the combined resources of many countries.

A perfect example of this type of garden is to be seen in the restoration of the various gardens at Mount Vernon, the home of George Washington. Developed in the closing years of the eighteenth century, both mansion and grounds are characterized by the most gracious dignity and careful design. Advantage was taken of everything that was known of good gardening.

The kitchen garden is surrounded by a high brick wall against which are espaliered fruit trees. There are two large brick dipping wells as focal points in the long axis of the garden. With simple accuracy this garden has been reproduced with the utmost consideration for the household needs in the time that it was first made. It holds an alluring collection of healing simples, culinary and pot herbs, and horticultural treasures. Garden herbs and vegetables are planted in borders in the geometrically arranged beds with thought for charming color combinations, textures and garden scents. Box, once set out as cuttings for future use in the flower garden, has grown into thickets.

There is no doubt that Washington drew freely upon his agricultural library for plant lists and horticultural directions. He owned both of Philip Miller's works on gardening, the Dictionary and the Calendar, printed in England, 1735, Batty Langley's "New Principles of Gardening," 1728. These books became important guides in late Colonial gardening. As a result the magnificent gardens built around the great estates of that period show close resemblance to the well remembered gardens of the homeland.

Old Roses for the Herb Garden

These came into our American gardens from the Continent and England during the eighteenth and nineteenth centuries. Here they were cherished with a love inspired by no modern hybrid today.

With the passing of the lovely Colonial garden of the nineteenth century many varieties were "lost." Others have remained hidden in the oblivion of overgrowth and weeds until their unsurpassed fragrance betrayed them to the collector of these sweet old roses.

It is heartening to think that they are now being sought out by ardent rose collectors of Europe, who gladly return them to their homelands. Calypso, the brilliant rose-pink noisette, was found a hundred years ago in a Pennsylvania garden. From a derelict garden in the old South was discovered "Couleur de Cuive," catalogued for American gardens in 1811. The Portland roses were believed extinct until someone found them in old American gardens.

Collectors of flower paintings know the exquisite "velvet rose" so frequently seen in arrangements. Someone found it in an old Long Island garden, where it had been growing for nearly two centuries.

In 1768, New England sent to the mother country rose d'amour, *flora plena*. I think that this was a double form of our own wild pink rose.

Even if the herb garden is not built around some delightful old home, there should be a place for a few old roses, and the following list is merely suggestive. (Read Miss Keays' story of the "Old Roses.")

Rosa alba and *Rosa rubra* are the white and red roses of the old world and perhaps we know their tall, flower-laden bushes as the "cottage rose." A pinkish variety is known as "the maiden's blush." *R. moschata* is the musk rose and its variety, *R. cinnamomea*, is the little pink cinnamon rose of country roadsides and tumbling stone walls. *Rosa centifolia*, cabbage rose or the "Red Provence," with its great heads of doubled petals, is the pink rose of country gardens, as is its close relation, the old moss rose. *Rosa damascena*, the damask rose, is often the last bush to leave the abandoned farm, but it is seldom that we see its red and white striped variety, the rose of Lancaster and York. *R. gallica*, the French or apothecaries' rose, has many varieties.

The collector of old roses knows that for him no hunting of antiques has the appeal that has this search for the "roses of yesterday."

List of a Few Sweet-Scented Geraniums Available in Nurseries Today

They are of the lemon-scented, mint-scented, rose-scented and aromatic varieties. Besides these there are species with decided fruit and spice scent. At present the nomenclature is greatly confused.

Pelargonium capitatum—Larger-leaved than rose; strong scent.
P. citriodorum, Prince of Orange—Strong orange fragrance.
P. Clorinda—An old favorite. Flowers freely.
P. crispum—True finger bowl geranium.
P. crispum, Prince Rupert—Yellow variegated.
P. denticulatum, Dr. Livingston—Foliage deeply cut; pleasant fragrance.
P. filtrum, Mrs. Taylor—Lovely dark red flower, leaves deeply cut.
P. graveolens—True rose geranium.
P. graveolens, Lady Plymouth—The variegated rose geranium.
P. limoneum, Lady Mary—Blooms freely. Sweet, spicy scent.
P. mellissimum—Balm. Large, hairy leaves, much like the rose geranium. Flowers pink and showy.
P. odoratissimum—Nutmeg or apple scented. Small round leaves, soft grayish. Very sweet.
P. Pretty Polly—Almond scented.
P. quercifolium, Fair Ellen—An oakleaf variety.
P. quercifolium, Oakleaf—Round-lobed leaf with dark center. A fine trailing type.
P. Shottesham Pet—Filbert scented. A lovely plant, yellow-green and soft-leaved.
P. tomentosum—Peppermint geranium. Large, dark green, velvety leaves.

One or two collectors in New England have discovered over fifty varieties of fragrant geraniums with a zeal which compares entertainingly with that of earlier interest when these plants were first introduced into England and thence to us.

Herbs Mentioned in Colonial Records Before 1700
(From "Gardens of Colony and State")

Balm, belury, chives, clary, five finger, hyssop, lovage, mint, mustard (single white), peppergrass, sage, sweet marjoram, summer savory, thyme, tarragon and wormwood.

Shrubs Mentioned Before 1700

Privet (primworth, skedge, skedgewith), flowering peach, double persica, white thorn (*Crataegus*).

"Flowering currant" not known. The well-known, old-fashioned shrub with fragrant yellow flowers (*Ribes odoratum*) was introduced from the Middle West at a later time.

Plants Known to Have Been Grown in Colonial Gardens After 1700

(From "Gardens of Colony and State")

ANEMONES
CARNATION, CLOVE PINK, *Dianthus caryophyllus*
COLUMBINE, *Aquilegia*—Not the new long-spurred varieties.
CROWN IMPERIAL, *Fritillaria imperialis*
DAFFODILS, *Narcissus poeticus* and *Narcissus Von Sion*
EVENING STOCKS, *Mathiola bicornis*
GILLIFLOWER STOCKS, *Mathiola incana*
GRAPE FLOWER or MUSCARY, *Muscari botryoides*
HOLLYHOCK, *Althaea rosea*
HOUSELEEK, *Sempervivum tectorum*
MARTAGON LILY, *Lilium martagon*
MARYGOLD, both single and double, *Calendula officinalis*
MOONWORT, SATTIN FLOWER, *Lunaria annua*
PRIMROSE, *Primula vulgaris*
ROSES, many old varieties.
SCARLET CROSS, *Lychnis chalcedonica*
SEDUM, several sorts.
STAR OF BETHLEHEM, *Ornithogalum umbellatum*
SUNFLOWER, *Helianthus annuus*
SWEETBRIAR, *Rosa rubiginosa*
TULIPS, many varieties.
VIOLETS, three kinds.
YELLOW DAY LILY, *Hemerocallis flava*

This list is far from complete, but it may serve as a "start" for the Colonial gardener.

Between 1700 and 1750, we read of "Amaranth, Bachelor's Buttons, Bell flowers (*Campanula*), Candy Tuff (*Iberis amara*), Devil in a Bush (*Nigella*), Flower de Luce (*Iris*), Fraxinella (*Dictamnus fraxinella*), Jacob's Ladder (*Polemonium*), Lilacs (deep blue, white, purple, and Persian), Lily of the Valley, Peonies (white and red), Periwinkle, Southernwood, Spiderwort (*Tradescantia*), and the Striped Scotch Rose."

In 1736 we read that Thomas Hancock of Boston ordered "yew trees, hollies, yew in the rough, for topiary work."

No reference was made to box having been grown in the North before 1800.

Between 1750 and 1800, mention is made of Persian iris, double China pinks, double larkspur, and snapdragons; in 1734, corn flag and gladioli; in 1763, the double white daffodil and double hyacinth, as well as oleanders and tuberose.

CHAPTER III

A GARDEN OF WILD HERBS

JUST when did the making of "wild gardens" become one of our present day horticultural pastimes? When for one reason or the other did our native and introduced simples become cultivated habitants of the yard?

We know that in all of the early settlements of America the Colonists planted near their homes medicinal and otherwise useful plants where, out of reach of Indian arrows, they could be conveniently gathered when needed.

We find today the descendants of these vitally important simples coming up year after year through the grass and weeds of these old homesteads, even though all other signs of former occupancy have vanished. We know them well: thoroughwort, Joe Pye weed, bloodroot, coltsfoot, Bouncing Bet.

Lacking the drug shop and its modern array, Colonial housewives were quick to find real or imaginary healing in the roots, stems, leaves and flowers of wild plants, which bore a resemblance to those well-known simples of their homeland.

In strange surroundings, they found American elder, *Sambucus canadensis*. It was not unlike its English cousin, *Sambucus nigra*, and they found its flowers made the same soothing tea and salve.

Under the folded early leaves of wild ginger, they saw and smelled its pungent roots, which reminded them of their own English asarabacca and served the same medicinal purpose in easing cramping pains and also for use as a snuff.

On the seacoast grew wild samphire, *Salicornia herbacea*, whose brittle stems made the same salty pickle as did its English cousin *Crithmum maritimum*, the true samphire of the English cliffs, washed by the same sea.

It must have been an exciting adventure, exploring the resources of these new lands, and bits of historical fact and fiction accumulate to make our wild gardens more than horticultural pastimes.

John Bartram's botanic garden near Philadelphia was founded in 1730. Through its records runs the story of those indefatigable plant explorers and botanists who defied privation and discouragements to bring into cultivation so many now familiar herbs, shrubs and trees which before 1800 were found only in the wilds.*

The smoke tree, *Rhus cotinus*, has been in cultivation since 1656; *Robinia hispida*, rose acacia, since 1758; and the flowering quince was introduced into Colonial gardens in 1790.

Then in 1784 we hear of clethra, azaleas, kalmias and halesia, the silver bell tree.

It was discovered that the bark of flowering dogwood, *Cornus florida*, made a tea as curative in intermittent fever as the South American quinine.

For just how long this interest was purely herbal is a matter of conjecture, but it is most probable that at first all introductions were made to serve some medicinal or otherwise economic use.

"*Close to the dome a garden shall be joined*
A fit employment for a studious mind;
In our vast woods, whatever simples grow,
Whose virtues none, or none but Indians know,
Within the confines of this garden brought,
To rise with added lustre shall be taught;
Then culled with judgment, each shall yield its juice,
Saliferous balsam to the sick man's use;
A longer date of life mankind shall boast,
And Death shall mourn her ancient sceptre lost."
    —"Bachelor's Hall" by George Webb, published 1731.

---

* "Peter Kalm's Travels in North America," by A. D. Benson, gives us a picture of our America of 1750.

Just where this garden was made is not known. It may be imaginary, or it may have belonged to the secretary of William Penn, James Logan. But the manuscript is of historic interest because it verifies a very early interest in the making of "wild gardens."

The modern development of large estates includes in the landscaping plan delightful opportunities for this kind of gardening.

There is such a planting in Milton, Massachusetts, which, each year, is open to all who delight in seeing the native herbs in their natural setting. Here is a twisting brook with a miniature cliff and its waterfall, a quiet pond, the shade of great evergreens, and the sifting sunlight through deciduous trees, low woodlands and open fields, all making perfect habitats for the wild things.*

Suggestions for Native Plants of Herb Interest, Easily Cultivated in the "Wild Garden"

These species include plants that, though originally introduced, have long been thought of as wild.

For swampy woodlands, edges of ponds, bogs with acid, peaty soil.

AMERICAN GOAT'S RUE, *Tephrosia virginiana*—This species needs loose, gravelly soil and dryer spots than the European goat's rue. The offensive smell of the bruised plant is characteristic of both.

BALMONY or TURTLE HEAD, *Chelone glabra*—A tall herb with showy rose-tinged flowers. A valuable "jaundice herb." The leaves of the red turtle head, *Chelone lyoni*, made a healing skin ointment.

BLUE FLAG, *Iris versicolor*

BLUE VERVAIN, SIMPLERS' JOY, *Verbena hastata*—An emetic herb used from earliest times in Colonial medicine.

---
*The Herbarist, 1935, Publication Herb Society of America, "Some Herbs From the Old World and the New That Will Grow in New England," Alice T. Whitney.

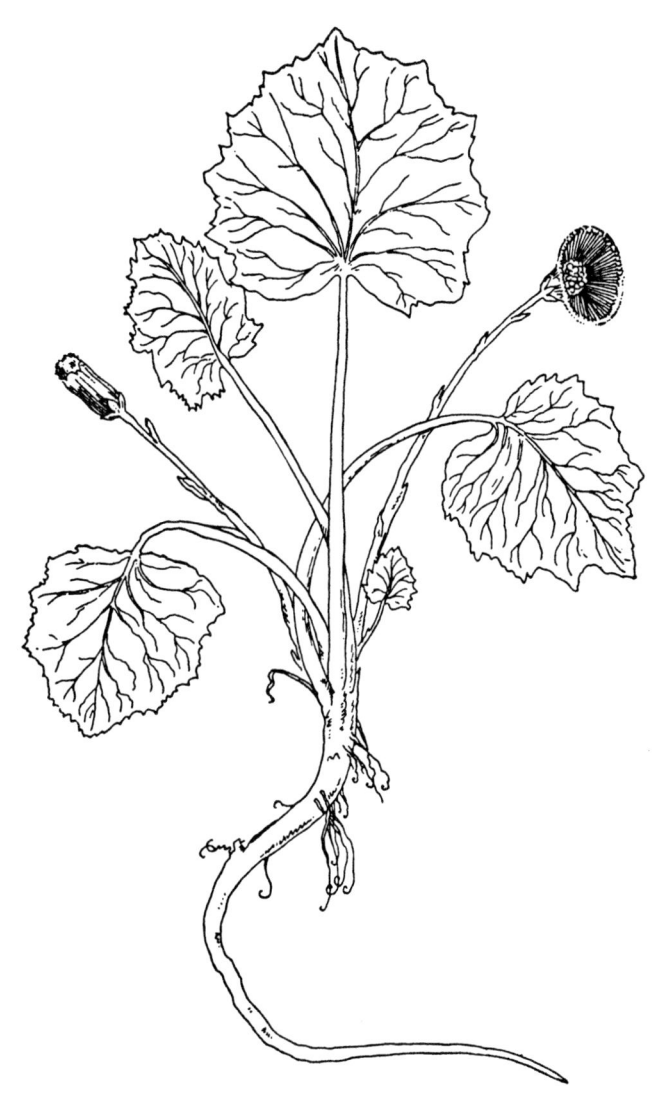

Tussilago farfara Coltsfoot: from Fuchs *Herbal*, 1542.

BONESET, or THOROUGHWORT, *Eupatorium perfoliatum*

BOWMAN'S ROOT, *Gillenia trifoliata*—A most attractive bush with white flowers. Likes moist thickets.

CENTAURY, *Centaurium umbellatum*—As to just which species was indicated in Anglo-Saxon therapy, we cannot be sure, but as its name, *Centum aurum*, implies, it was a "priceless cure worth a hundred gold pieces." It has pale purple flowers and is not a showy herb, and belongs to the gentian family. Note: This herb should not be confused with old-world garden herbs of the genus *Centaurea*, which belongs to the composite family. In this group are "Dusty Miller," *Centaurea cineraria*, a tender gray tomentose annual much used for borders in Victorian gardens, also bachelor's buttons, *C. cyanus*.

COLTSFOOT, *Tussilago farfara*

CULVER'S PHYSIC, *Veronicastrum virginicum*—A woody, showy herb with blue flowers.

GOAT'S RUE, *Galega officinalis*—A bushy legume with white pea-like flowers and foliage. Its leaves and stems were used, and perhaps are to this day, to bring on profuse sweating in fevers.

GOLDTHREAD, *Coptis trifolia*—Its delicate golden roots are medicinal.

GREEN HELLEBORE, *Veratrum viride*—Showy wrinkled leaves and yellow-green sprays of flowers; a bitter medicinal root.

HERB O' GRACE, *Verbena officinalis*—Its legendary history and its numerous medicinal virtues warrant it a place in our herb garden even if its most uninteresting weedy appearance and insignificant small flowers do not.

JOE PYE WEED, *Eupatorium purpurium*

LABRADOR TEA, *Ledum groenlandicum*—A fragrant, low-growing evergreen shrub, with clustered white flowers. Its leaves made the Revolutionary tea.

MARSH MARIGOLD (sometimes wrongly called "cowslips"), *Caltha palustris*—Its yellow-gold flowers are seen in early spring standing up out of icy pools. The young plants are eaten as pot herbs, a silly transgression of good conservation. (Green buds are said to be poison.)

PURPLE LOOSESTRIFE, *Lythrum salicaria*—As its common name implies, the whole plant was efficacious in releasing the stress of disordered minds.

SABATIA—Several species of this genus belonging to the gentian family are of herb interest. None of them transplant readily from the salt marshes where they are biennial or annual, but all are very beautiful with rose pink or white flowers and, once established, will give great pleasure.

SWEET FLAG, *Acorus calamus*—Perennial. Thick, creeping root used for the sweet-flag candy of Shaker fame.

YELLOW FLAG, *Iris pseudacorus*—This herb is thought to have been the "gladiolus" of mediæval herb lists.

In ponds and in sphagnum bogs, there are three herbs of great medicinal interest and loveliness which may be easily introduced by seeds.

PITCHER PLANT, *Sarracenia purpurea*—This is a noted insectivorus plant of our peat bogs. The seedlings straddle the sphagnum and in a year make bronze and green clumps of pitcher-shaped leaves from which rise in midsummer fragrant, nodding, purple-red blossoms. The whole plant was an Indian remedy which lessened the pitting resulting from smallpox.

SUNDEW, *Drosera*—Several species. In the sunshine, the slender stems of its white flowers rise above the leaves. The latter are covered with viscid tentacles which fold over unwary mosquitoes. All species are still used as a whooping-cough remedy.

WATER LILY, *Nymphaea odorata*—It is not easy to think of this exquisite flower as a medicinal herb, but such it was and belongs in the herb garden.

Where the real woodland begins, and in semi-shade, a number of decorative herbs will find a place.

AGRIMONY, *Agrimonia striata*—Its familiar yellow wands and

rosettes of soft, reddish-veined leaves are attractive. An ancient Anglo-Saxon medicinal.

ALUM ROOT, *Heuchera americana*

ANISE GOLDENROD, *Solidago odora*—One of the favorite "tea herbs" of Revolutionary days.

BLACK SNAKEROOT or BLACK COHOSH, *Cimicifuga racemosa*

BLUE LOBELIA, *Lobelia syphilitica*

CANADA LILY, *Lilium canadense*

CARDINAL FLOWER, *Lobelia cardinalis*—Bright red flowers.

CELANDINE, *Chelidonum majus*—Ancient medicinal herb.

COLIC ROOT, *Aletris farinosa*

GOLDEN SEAL, *Hydrastis canadensis*—Cultivated today in the United States for its medicinal root.

JACK IN THE PULPIT, *Arisaema tryphyllum*

MAY APPLE, *Podophyllum peltatum*—Edible fruits. A medicinal herb in use today.

RED BANEBERRY, *Actaea rubra*—Poisonous red berries.

WHITE BANEBERRY, *Actaea alba*—Poisonous white berries.

WHITE SNAKEROOT, *Eupatorium rugosum*

WILD SARSAPARILLA, *Aralia nudicaulis*—Woody, aromatic roots.

WILD SWEET CICELY, *Osmorhiza longistylis, O. claytoni*—Are not unlike the garden sweet cicely, with lacy umbels of white flowers and fernlike leaves. The roots are sweet to the taste and fragrant when dry.

In the carpet of the same woodland, are other humble green herbs which love the loose, rich leaf mold.

BIRTH ROOT, *Trillium*—Several species of herb interest.

BLOODROOT, *Sanguinaria canadensis*—The thick, blood-red root stalks have been used from earliest days for whooping cough and other bronchial affections.

CLUB MOSSES, *Lycopodium*—There are several species of these little evergreen plants which belong to the great order of non-flowering plants, and reproduce themselves by spores instead of seeds. They are the little "creeping evergreens" which have been used medicinally for centuries. The clouds of spores in their "clubs" make a dusting powder used like "talcum." Because of the water-repellent properties of these spores, the apothecary uses them to coat pills.

FALSE MITREWORT, *Tiarella cordifolia*—Likes the richest of rocky woods.

DWARF GINSENG, GROUND NUT, *Panax trifolium*

(The Chinese herb whose root is so highly prized is *Panax schinseng*.)

HEPATICA, *Hepatica triloba*—Grows well in woods under oaks and maples.

LESSER CELANDINE or PILEWORT, *Ranunculus ficaria*—Small light gold flowers with shining leaves.

MAIDENHAIR FERN, *Adiantum pedatum*—A cooling fever herb.

PARTRIDGE BERRY, SQUAW BERRY, *Mitchella repens*—An Indian remedy used to relax muscles and ease childbirth pains.

POLYPODY, ROCK FERN, *Polypodium vulgare*—Clings in mats to the rocks.

PRINCE'S PINE, PIPSISSEWA, *Chimaphila umbellata*—Root used for rheumatism.

SHIN LEAF, PYROLY, *Pyrola rotundifolia*—Used in rheumatic fevers.

SQUIRREL CORN, *Dicentra canadensis*—Needs pockets of rich woodland earth and wet rocks.

WILD GINGER, *Asarum canadense*

If we have dry pasture land in the wild garden, we shall probably find numerous wild herbs already established.

BROOM BUDS, *Cytisus scoparius*—A woody yellow flowered herb, an early escape from gardens in Salem, Massachusetts.

CHECKERBERRY OF WINTERGREEN, *Gaultheria procumbens*

MEADOW-SWEET, *Spiraea salicifolia*—The Shakers used great quantities in brewing their botanic beer, for it was sweet in flavor and saved sugar.

MOUNTAIN MINT, *Pycnanthemum*—All species are aromatic, bushy herbs which make tonic medicinal teas.

NEW JERSEY TEA, *Ceanothus americanus*

STEEPLE BUSH, *Spiraea tomentosa*

TANSY, *Tanacetum vulgare*

TEASEL, *Dipsacus fullonum*—Biennial herbs with prickly, recurved spines on their lovely flower heads, which are used to comb velvet, thereby giving this herb its old-country name, "Brushes and Combs." The opening of the florets on the flower cone of this herb is one of the lovely phenomena in nature.

WILD PENNYROYAL, *Hedeoma pulegioides*

WOAD WAXEN, *Genista tinctoria*

WOOD BETONY, LOUSEWORT, *Pedicularis canadensis*—A famous herb of our dry woodlands.

YARROW, *Achillea millefolium*—Will be everywhere whether we like it or not, but let it stay, for its early history is honorable.

For a more complete list of herbs for "wild gardens," see the new edition (1942) of "Standardized Plant Names," prepared for the American Joint Committee on Horticultural Nomenclature by its Editorial Committee, Harlan P. Kelsey and William A. Dayton, J. Horace McFarland Co., Publishers.

CHAPTER IV

A FEW IMPORTANT HERB FAMILIES AND THEIR GENERA

IT IS perplexing to choose from among several hundred plant families, those few which might be called "herb families," for in the plant world there are not many families that do not count among their members some herb of economic use to man.

The following families are listed because they either include a large number of herbs or a few of importance to the herb gardener. Botanically, for convenience in classification, the families, as they are called, are divided into genera, each of which we know as a *genus*.

The genus may include few or many kinds of plants called species, grouped thus because they have obvious similarity.

Thus the plant family of the LABIATAE, popularly called the mint family, includes the genus *Mentha*. But not all "mints," popularly so called, are *mints* to the careful botanist, who may confine that term to the genus *Mentha* which includes the *true mints*.

The genus *Mentha* is divided into a fairly large number of species, of which *Mentha spicata*, the common spearmint, is one, and the crisp-leaved plant so like it otherwise in smell and flower is *Mentha spicata crispata*.

Plants of a species which vary from the type in one or two minor but constant differences constitute a *variety* with an additional variety name.

And what herb gardener has not been confronted by an array of *Mentha* seedlings appearing in his garden which show, besides resemblances, bewildering variations from the parent type species, *Mentha spicata?*

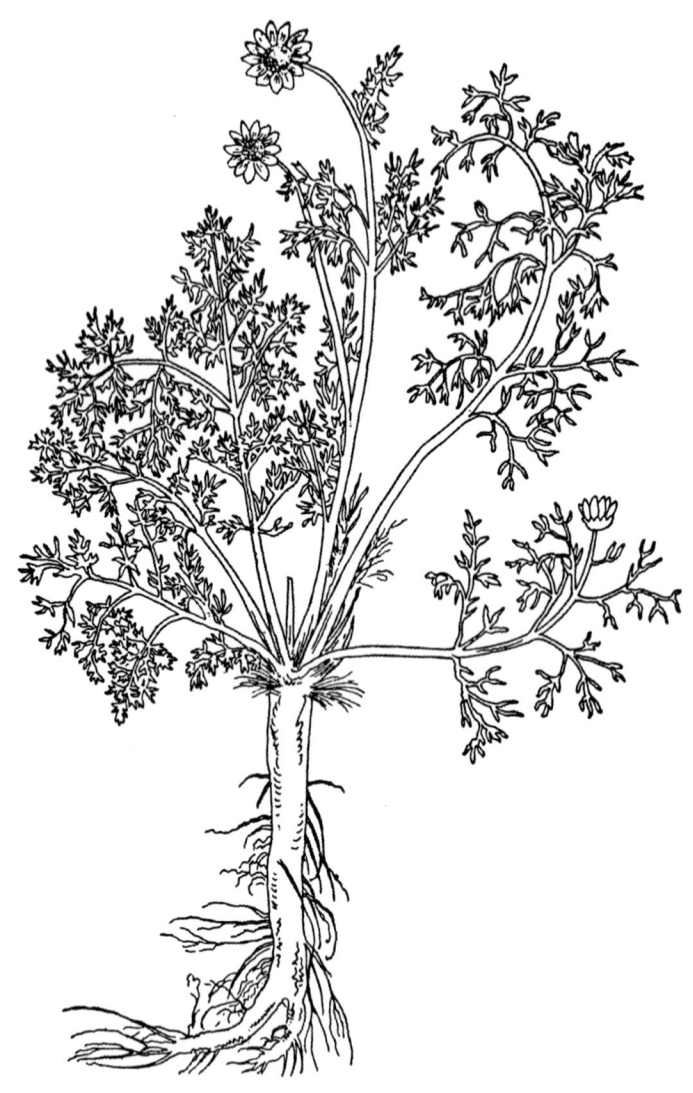

Chrysanthemum cineriaefolium Pyrethrum: from Fuchs, 1542.

There is more confusion among popular names in the herbs than in any other group of plants. From earliest days the country or folk name often designated its special medicinal or other local use.

Viola tricolor, our familiar little Johnny-jump-up, counts over forty folk names in English vernacular alone. Some are of obvious origin, others suggestive of entertaining research.*

Likewise to add to the nomenclatorial confusion are synonyms for the same species, though it is botanical custom to accept, if possible, the name first given the plant.

Mentha viridis is the same plant as *Mentha spicata*. Both are spearmint.

Another example is the common magenta-flowered *wild basil* which in its herbal history of some three thousand years has been called by herbalist and botanist *Thymus, Calamintha* and *Clinopodium*. At present it seems to have found a permanent nomenclatorial home in the genus *Satureia* (savory).

Frequently two or more different plants may have the same common name. And here alone the correct scientific name of the botanist can straighten out the tangle. "Queen of the Meadow," spoken of in herbals, is *Spiraea ulmaria*, a well known medicinal herb. But the American colonist knew as "Queen of the Meadow" another medicinal simple, the purple *Eupatorium purpureum*, also known as Joe Pye weed. Opinions will differ as to which herb family is most important.

The BORAGE FAMILY, BORAGINACEAE, includes a number of herbs of almost forgotten medicinal value which are now loved garden favorites. They are mucilaginous, rather weedy, slightly bitter, and the roots of some of the plants yield a red dye.

In the herb garden are these genera:

ALKANET, *Anchusa* HELIOTROPE, *Heliotropium*
BORAGE, *Borago* LUNG-WORT, *Pulmonaria*
COMFREY, *Symphytum* MERTENSIA
FORGET-ME-NOT, *Myosotis*

---

*See "Dictionary of Plant Names," Gerth van Wijk.

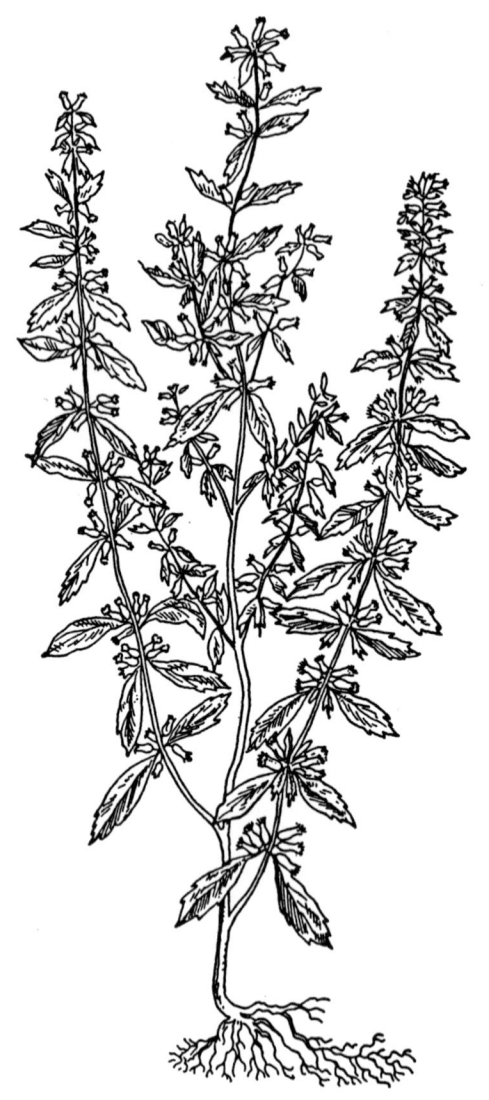

Hedeoma pulegioides American Pennyroyal: from Barton's Medical Botany of the United States, 1818.

The COMPOSITAE FAMILY is the largest plant family in the world. Its plants are called COMPOSITAE because of the flower heads, which are made up of closely clustered florets.

The COMPOSITAE are easily recognized for the tiny flowers are arranged in a close head on the receptacle, which is merely the enlarged top of the stem that bears them. Sometimes there are bright ray flowers on the outside of these heads as in feverfew, common daisy, sunflower and elecampane. Or the heads may be composed of all ray flowers as in the Chaucer daisy, dandelion and chicory.

Tansy and costmary have buttonlike heads of closely packed tubular florets.

This family of COMPOSITAE has more than a thousand genera, including plants of great beauty and many herbs with interesting histories: goldenrod, aster, thoroughwort, coltsfoot. It includes pot herbs, insecticides and medicinals.

The genus *Chrysanthemum* is one of the largest in this family. Many of its species have been brought to high horticultural development and several are of economic importance as herbs. Pyrethrum powder is made from the flower head of *Chrysanthemum cineriaefolium*.

Used for centuries as pot herbs are lettuce, thistle, salsify, dandelion and chicory.

Once a medicinal, now a terrible pest, is ragweed or "bitter weed," of the genus *Ambrosia*. Ragweed is also called Roman wormwood* and should not be confused with *sweet ambrosia*, an old-time favorite of our herb gardens, which is also called Roman wormwood, and belongs to an entirely different family, the CHENOPODS.

Perhaps the most representative genera of COMPOSITAE in our modern herb garden are:

CHAMOMILE, *Anthemis*   LAVENDER COTTON, *Santolina*
ELECAMPANE, *Imula*   MARIGOLD, *Calendula*

---

*Perhaps the name "Roman wormwood" properly belongs to *Artemisia pontica*, the low-growing feathery herb sometimes used for edgings.

MUGWORT, or WORMWOOD, TARRAGON, SOUTHERNWOOD, *Artemisia*
SAFFLOWER, *Carthamus*
SWEET MARY, *Chrysanthemum*
YARROW, *Achillea*

The GOOSEFOOT FAMILY, or *Chenopodiaceae*, includes a curious group of herbs, mostly annuals, with insignificant yellowish-green flowers and succulent stems. Besides *Beta* (beet) many weed pests like pig weed are "herb genera" of varied interest, as:

AMBROSIA or JERUSALEM OAK, *Chenopodium*
GOOD KING HENRY, *Blitum*
ORACH, *Atriplex*
SAMPHIRE, *Crithmum*

The LILY FAMILY, LILIACEAE. The herbal histories of a few genera in this family are indicative of the transition of the herb as a plant of great medicinal importance to equally great prominence in the flower garden.

Lilium, which includes the Madonna lily, and *Convallaria*, lily-of-the-valley, scilla, yucca, and so many other plants of horticultural value, are now seldom even thought of as herbs.

Even though claimed by the florist, two genera remain of undeniable use in the herb garden today:

MEADOW SAFFRON, *Colchicum*   ONIONS, *Allium*

The MINT FAMILY, botanically known as the LABIATAE, from one of its flower characteristics, the two parted corolla with a lower lip, includes the largest number of aromatic herbs, and we recognize them as "mints" chiefly by their square stems, opposite leaves, and the pungent oil ducts.

Most of the members of this large family are natives of southern Europe and the eastern countries but they have adapted themselves and their economic uses to all climates of the civilized world.

Of the one hundred and fifty or more genera in this family commonly included in our herb gardens are:

BASIL, *Ocimum*
BEE BALM, *Monarda*
BUGLE, *Ajuga*
CALAMINT, *Calamintha*

A FEW IMPORTANT HERB FAMILIES AND THEIR GENERA 77

CATMINT, *Nepeta*
DEAD NETTLE, *Lamium*
GERMANDER, *Teucrium*
HOREHOUND, *Marrubium*
HYSSOP, *Hyssopus*
LAVENDER, *Lavandula*

LEMON BALM, *Melissa*
MARJORAM, *Origanum*
"MINTS," *Mentha*
ROSEMARY, *Rosmarinus*
SAVORY, *Satureia*
THYME, *Thymus*

The MUSTARD FAMILY, called CRUCIFERAE because the four spreading petals of its flowers form a Greek cross. In its two thousand or more genera are no poisonous plants. They are acrid herbs for the most part with spicy seeds which make famous condiments. Many herbs of this family have become weed pests though not so thought of in those bygone days when races depended on them for pot herbs and spice.

Sweet alyssum, wall flower and candytuft are well known ornamentals of the flower border, and sweet rocket.

Cabbage, kale and turnip are pot herbs which belong to the genus *Brassica*, a large and important group from whose species are being developed all manner of new varieties in the vegetable world. "Lady's Smocks," loved by Shakespeare, is *Cardamine*, a white-flowered mustard.

Woad, an ancient "dye herb," is *Isatis*.

In the herb garden we find also the genera:

HORSE RADISH, *Cochlearia armoracia*
PEPPER GRASS, *Lepidium*
SCURVY GRASS, *Cochlearia*

ST. BARBARA'S HERB or WINTER CRESS, *Barbarea*
WATER CRESS, *Nasturtium*

The PARSLEY FAMILY is important as an herb family. Its plants are called UMBELLIFERAE because the numerous small flowers are arranged in more or less flat heads called umbels. The leaves are often fernlike and decorative.

In this very large family, with nearly three hundred genera, are well-known garden favorites.

It has been, since Bible times, a family famous for the aromatic, oily seeds of its plants. Some of its members are valuable garden vegetables or pot herbs used since the beginning of man. Others are herbs of equally ancient history containing deadly poisonous properties.

The genera of the herb garden best known are:

ANGELICA, *Archangelica*
ANISE, *Pimpinella*
CARAWAY, *Carum*
CHERVIL, *Anthriscus*
CORIANDER, *Coriandrum*
CUMIN, *Cuminum*
DILL, *Anethum*
FENNEL, *Foeniculum*
LOVAGE, *Levisticum*
PARSLEY, *Petroselinum*
SWEET CICELY, *Myrrhis*

The PEA or PULSE FAMILY — LEGUMINOSAE — is so called from the legume-shaped seed pods. It is a very large and well-known family which includes the greatest number of forage plants, and also herbs of great economic importance, drugs, dyes, oils, etc.

No plant family has made greater or more decorative contributions to gardens and arboretums over the known world than the PULSE family.

In the herb garden we may find:

BROOM, *Cytisus*
BUR CLOVER, *Medicago*
CLOVER, *Trifolium*
FENUGREEK, *Trigonella foe-num-Graecum*
SWEET CLOVER, *Melilotus*
WOAD WAXEN, WHIN, *Genista*

The ROSE FAMILY, ROSACEAE, includes a few herbs which still hold for the modern herbalist the charm of their primitive lore, although the value of raspberry, strawberry and blackberry leaves as tonic or medicinal teas is not considered so important as in the day of the Boston Tea Party.

In the herb garden are found today:

BURNET, *Sanguisorba*
LADY'S MANTLE, *Alchemilla*
SWEETBRIAR ROSE, *Rosa*

See also a list of "Herbs for the Wild Garden" (page 64).

CHAPTER V

DOCTRINE OF SIGNATURES

"AND by the icon or image of every herb, man first found out their virtues. Modern writers laugh at them for it, but I wonder in my heart how the virtues of herbs came first to be known, if not by their signatures. The moderns have them from the writings of the ancients, — the ancients had no writings to have them from." — Culpepper.

"The English Physician and Herbal" is a thick little book, leather bound and crackling with age, which was written by Culpepper about 1653. It is full of quaint observations on plants, commentaries on their uses, and amusing satire. No description of his is complete without some explanation of the great influence of the planets and constellations under which all herbs were protected.

This courtly old English physician believed in the "Doctrin of Signitures," as had many herbalists before his day. Every herb, he argued, must tell to man by its form or leaves, stem or flowers, of what use it might be in curing his ills. No members of the family of the CRUCIFERAE with their crossed petals can by poison bring harm to man. The lungwort has spotted leaves which show that it is a curative plant for diseased or spotted lungs. Butter-and-eggs, buttercup and dandelions were jaundice herbs.

"Some (herbs) by experiment we see, whose names express their natures!" Garlic with its hollow stalk helps affections of the windpipe.

Prunella is carpenter's herb, for the flower is shaped like a bill-hook or a sickle. "In all the world is not a better wound herb as has often been prooved!"

Solomon's seal (*Polygonatum biflorum*) has seal-shaped scars on the root stalk. "Root excellent, good for to seal or close up wounds, broken bones, and such like. It soldereth and glues together bones in a very short space of time and very strangely, yea, though the bones be but slenderly and unhandsomely placed and wrapped up!"

"If any herbe infest the earth with its abundance let man heed its great virtues for his ills." Dandelion, plantain or white man's foot, yarrow, nettles.

Was the modern use of salacin for rheumatic fever first suggested in this old belief in the doctrine of signatures?

Salacin is found in the bark of the willow and the alder, which grow in damp places conducive to rheumatism. Therefore to these simple believers, why should not these herbs cure diseases caused by dampness?

In the philosophy of Henry Vaughan, the early seventeenth-century poet and mystic, is the thread of this Hermetic philosophy.

> *"The herb becomes the teacher*
> *Men stray after false goals*
> *when the herb he treads knows much, much more."*

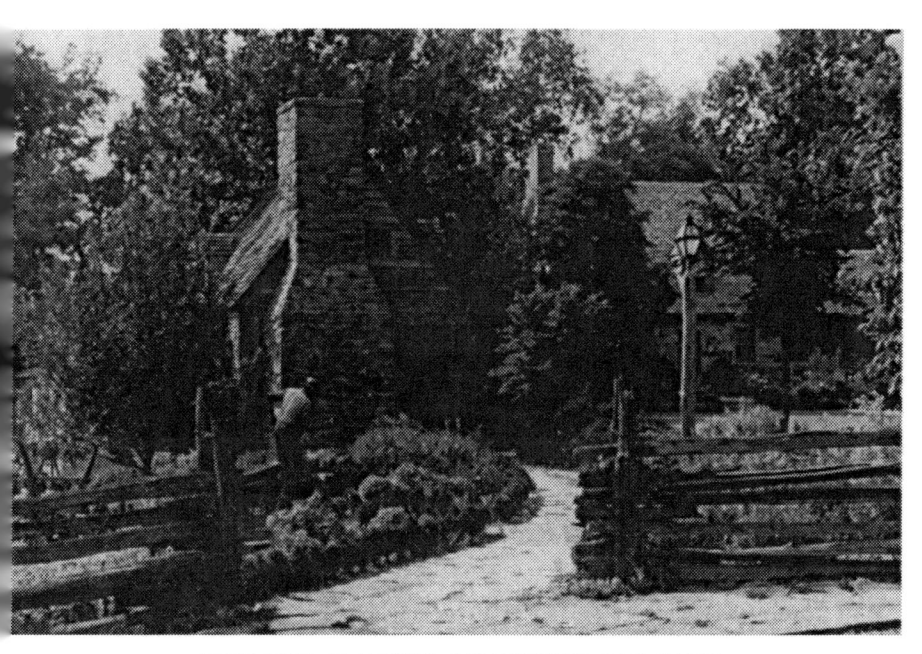

ENTRANCE PLANTING, WEATHERED OAK FARM
The herb house and old rail fence are consistently 18th Century Colonial.

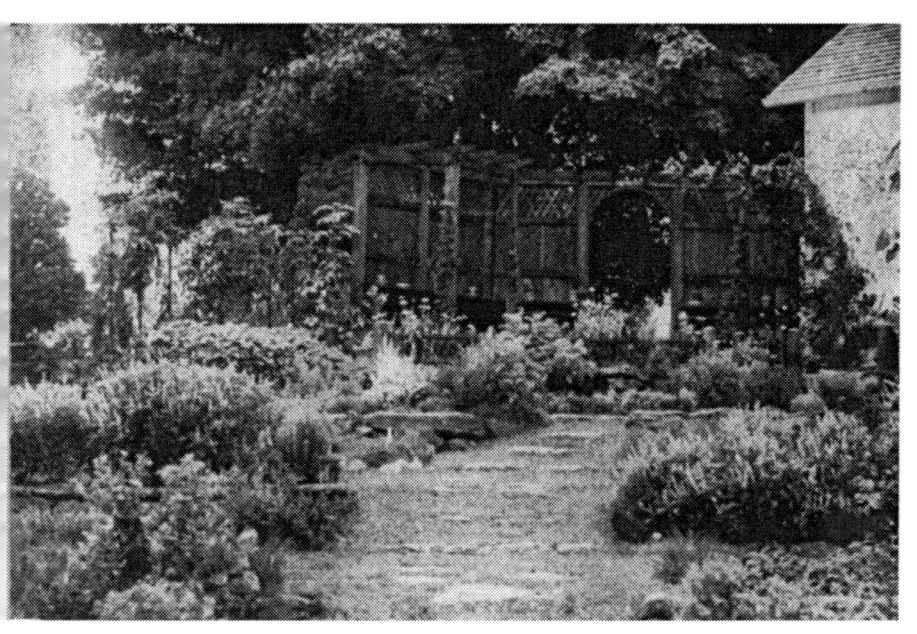

PATH PLANTING OF SWEET HERBS
Garden Centre, Stockbridge, Massachusetts. A lovely adaptation of an old custom. Fragrant herbs border the pathway to the door of the home.

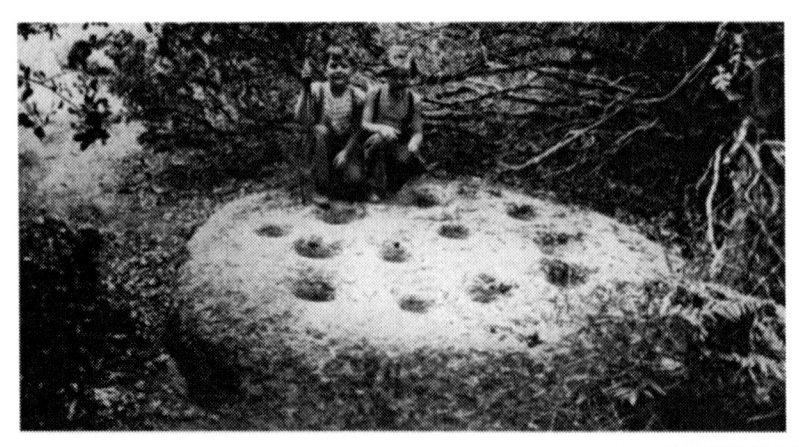

"APOTHECARY SHOP" OF THE NORTH AMERICAN INDIAN MEDICINE MAN
The thirteen mortars or holes, six or seven inches deep, were used for the different herb medicines. The stone is in San Jacinto State Park. Photo courtesy of Mrs. Percy Raymond.

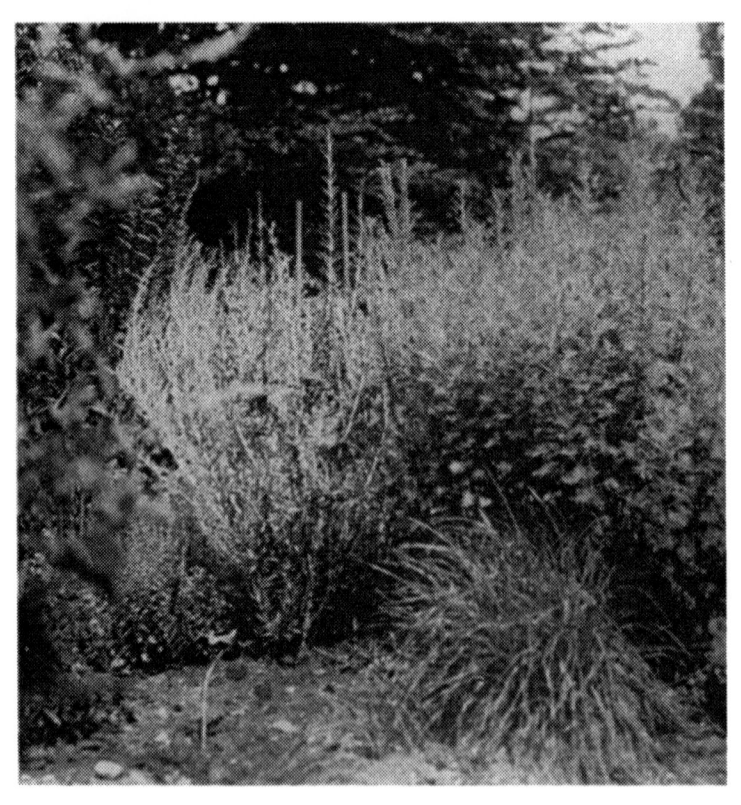

ROSEMARY, TALL MUGWORT AND CHIVES
Garden of Mr. and Mrs. Frederick Houghton, Milton, Massachusetts.

CHAPTER VI

MEDICINAL HERBS

THROUGH Colonial records and the numerous medical botanies published in the early years of the last century, we know much about the simples of America which were used for medicine and healing. Pioneer plant hunters from countries of Europe were primarily interested in the discovery of new drugs and the correspondence between them and the botanists and physicians of their various countries is most entertaining reading for us today. Monardes, the Bartrams, Kalm, Michaux, Rafinesque, Dr. Barton of Philadelphia and Dr. Bigelow of Boston all sent back their notes and the plants themselves to be tried out in the physic gardens of the Old World.

From 1800 until nearly the close of this century, the Shakers in New Lebanon, New York, as well as in their other communities were growing, drying and harvesting medicinal herbs for the market as one of their chief industries. A catalogue compiled in 1833, lists one hundred thirty-seven different herbs whose seeds, bark, root, leaves or flowers were bought and used by drug houses, pharmacists and physicians in both America and Europe.

In this catalogue, twelve extracts made from boneset, butternut, cicuta, dandelion, henbane, hop, garden and wild lettuce, deadly nightshade, garden nightshade and thorn apple, were advertised. Shaker ointments from marshmallow root, elder flowers, savin and stramonium were popular preparations. For their well ordered infirmaries, the sisters compounded rose and violet water for weary, aching heads, and ministered to the sick with their bilious, cephalic, and digestive pills, syrups of sarsaparilla, black cohosh and a host of other herbs. Their vegetable cough drops, made from

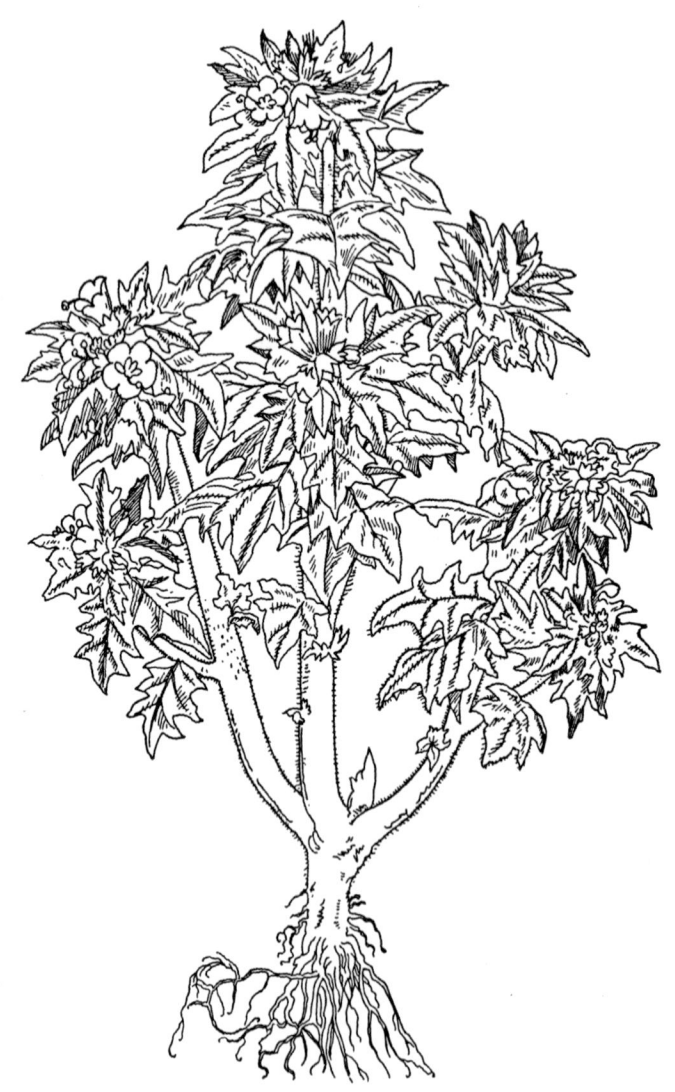

Hyocymus niger Henbane: from Fuchs Herbal, 1542.

horehound, flagroot, elecampane, slippery elm and lovage, were sold all over the country.

Wise in their herbal therapy as they were, many of these Shaker remedies hark back to almost the exact mediæval usage of the same herbs as recorded in Anglo-Saxon Apuleuis of the eleventh century.

The Shakers were thrifty conservationists, and though the brethren and sisters gathered much of their plant material from woods and fields, they saved many wild drug plants from extermination by cultivating them in their own gardens.

In the latter part of the last century commercial herb growing in America gradually flagged. There was a spasmodic renewal of interest during the first World War when experimental cultivation of a few needed medicinals, including digitalis ,belladonna and scopolia, achieved some success in meeting the scarcity of foreign imports.

However, competitive costs of foreign labor soon made American production of medicinal herbs unprofitable and the people of Europe were allowed to return to their ancient avocation of herb growing, harvesting and exporting.

Yet, in the ordering of human affairs, the pendulum always swings. Today the hostilities of a world at war and consequent curtailed imports of vitally necessary plant drugs are encouraging again commercial herb growing in the Americas. State universities with their great experiment stations, schools of pharmacognosy, drug houses and our federal government are announcing success in controlled cultivation of the necessary botanical drugs.

Peppermint and spearmint are grown in large acreage in the muck lands of Indiana and Wisconsin where they are reaped like hay and distilled for their oils.

Ephedra, a curious, flowerless plant from the arid soil of China, has been the oriental source of ephedrine for two thousand years and more. The three famous narcotics, scopolia, belladonna, henbane, which yield the powerful alkaloids of scopolamine, atropine and hyoscyamine, are cultivated in the warmer parts of the United States where they

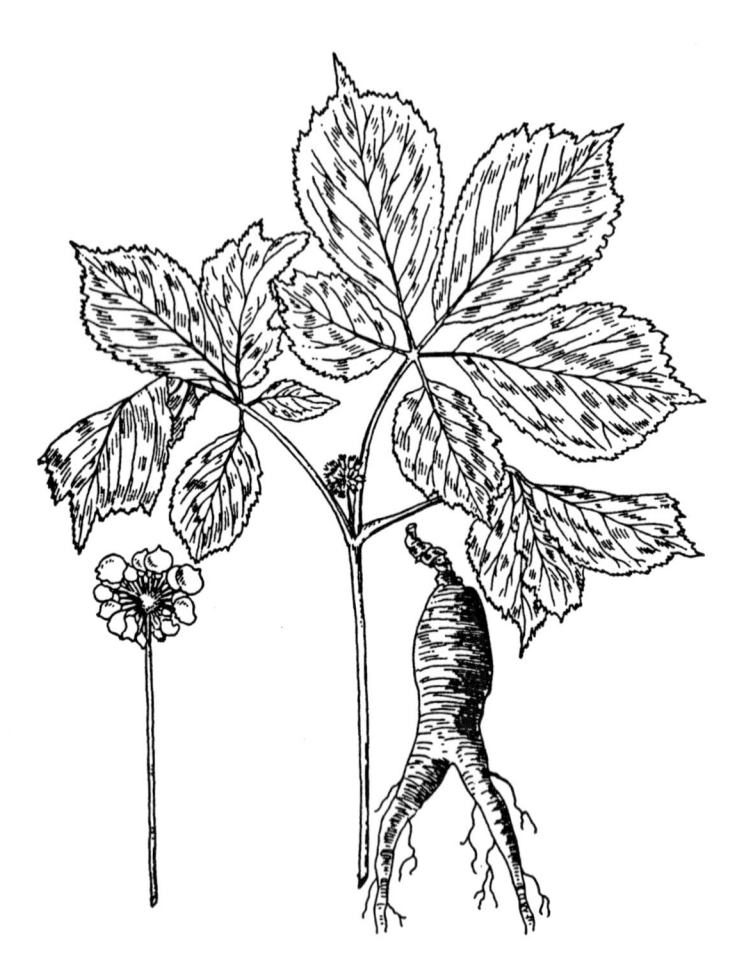

Panax quinquifolium American Ginseng: from Barton's Medical Botany of the United States, 1818.

MEDICINAL HERBS 85

have a long growing season. Aconite, larkspur, valerian, wormseed and a few others less well known, have also a strictly medicinal interest only to the pharmacist and physician. Their toxic principles render them unfit for food and they are poisonous in other than medicinal doses.

Swamp hellebore, burdock, tansy, wild arnica, jimson weed, have been brought in from the wild and grown for their volatile oils in small areas throughout the country.

From the bark of one of our native buckthorns comes the medicine *cascara sagrada*, but like so many other sources from which man has recklessly gathered his supplies this tree in the wild is now rarely found in quantity. Perhaps in time synthetic medicines will take the place of all these wild botanicals now collected for the drug trade and which are so rapidly nearing extermination.

Too often this unintelligent and useless gathering of fast disappearing woodland species is not warranted by their value to the trade. In this class are bethroot, goldthread, several orchids, pitcher plants, wild ginger, hepatica, aletris, arbutus, pasque flower, black snakeroot, blue cohosh, ginseng, puccoon and pulsatilla.

Books have been written on the cultivation of ginseng and golden seal in the United States where they have been profitable drug crops for a hundred years.

The story of American ginseng begins in 1714 when a missionary in China sent home a description of that miracle herb, Chinese ginseng (*Panax schinseng*), and recorded his belief that its counterpart might be found in the more northern woodlands of America. After long searching a plant was found near Montreal in 1716 by an Indian missionary, Father Lafitau. It was *Panax quinquefolium*, the American ginseng, so nearly like its Chinese cousin in appearance of the roots and its properties that the Chinese lost no time in accepting it, and thus was the ginseng trade established in America.

Of three hundred or more families of flowering plants in the world, about seventy include drug plants among their species, and these are exclusive of medicinal ferns and club mosses.

Three of these families perhaps most familiar to the layman and gardener are the night shade (*Solanaceae*) which gives us henbane, datura, tobacco, belladonna, and the "drowsy mandragora" of classic fame. The buttercup family (*Ranunculaceae*) is renowned for its poisonous watery and acrid juices and includes the hellebores, veratrums, baneberry, aconite, larkspur and pulsatilla. Best known in the figwort family (*Scrophulariaceae*) is digitalis, the foxglove which yields the medicinal alkaloid for which, as yet, no substitute has been found.

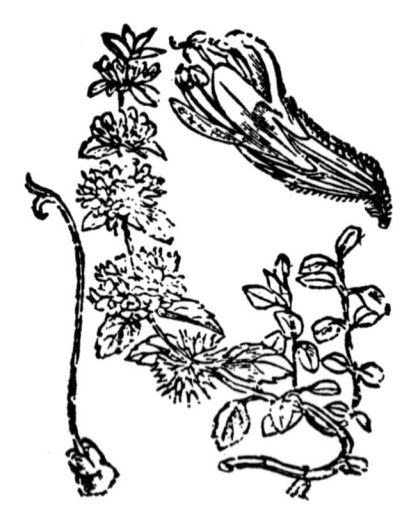

PENNYROYAL
M. Pulegium L.

All illustrations of Mentha from "British Flora," L. Reeve & Co.

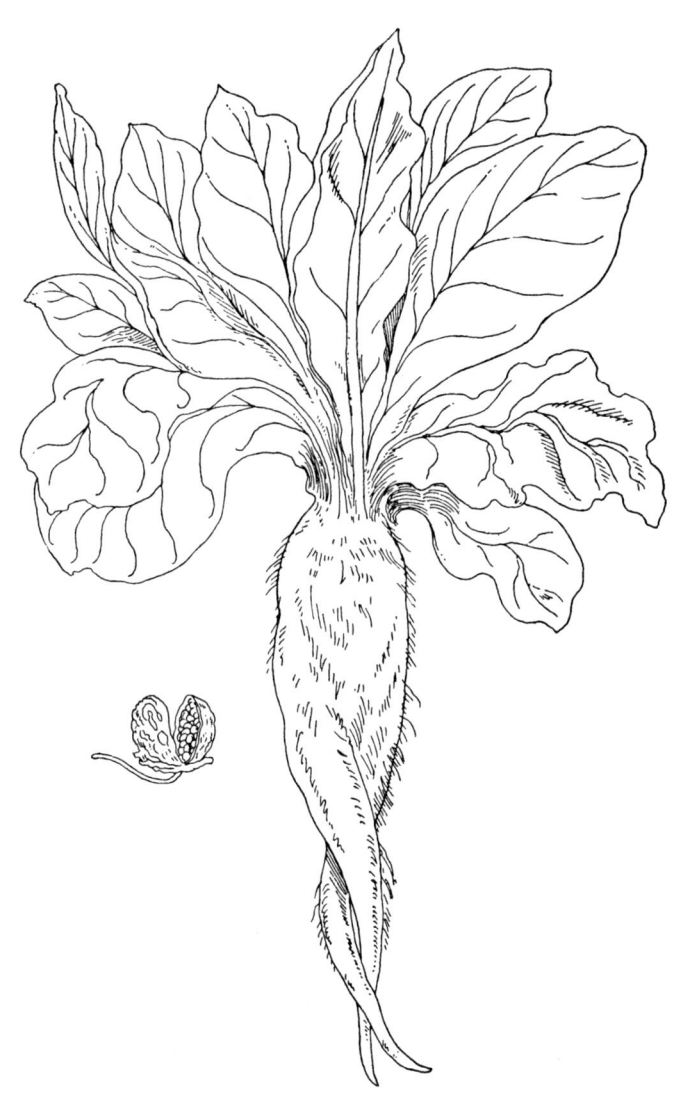

Mandragora autumnalis Mandrake: from Fuchs Herbal, 1542.

CHAPTER VII

GENERAL HORTICULTURAL DIRECTIONS FOR HERB GARDENS

"NOW it behooves any one who desires to be a skillful herbalist to be present when the herbs first shoot out of the earth, when they are fully grown, and when they begin to fade. For he who is only present at the budding of the herb, cannot know it when full grown, nor can he who hath examined a full grown herb, recognize it when it has just appeared above the ground!" — DIOSCORIDES.

Nearly all our sweet herbs were originally natives of Southern Europe and the Orient. Thymes and marjorams were known and used in the Mediterranean countries centuries before the Christian era. Angelica, yarrow and artemisia are found in the northern countries. Palestine and Smyrna are the homes of cumin, coriander, anise and lavender.

Horticulturally we can best treat herbs in our modern gardens by giving consideration to their native habitats. Generally speaking, they need warmth, sunlight, air, and for the most part a poor, well-drained, gravelly soil. They need lime or a "sweet" soil with an overbalance on the alkaline side, but in varying proportions. Burnet and rue thrive on the chalk cliffs of England; peppermint in the peat of Michigan.

Specific directions for the growing of different herbs are given in the discussion of "Herbs for Modern Gardens" (see page 141). The following experiences are personal.

Soil for the seed bed of herbs is made by sifting compost, one part; sand, two parts; loam, one part. I use fine window screening, and bake the soil for an hour to destroy fungus spores.

The compost I use happens to be from the rotten heart

GENERAL HORTICULTURAL DIRECTIONS FOR HERB GARDENS 89

of an old apple tree, which makes a rather richer growing medium for the seedlings than is necessary; however this saves time for, if the seedlings are not sown too thickly, this makes a growing mixture sufficient to carry them along without having to have them "pricked out" twice.

Herb seedlings germinate as in other groups of plants, some quickly, some slowly. It is at least three weeks before rosemary appears, and if I have not thoroughly sterilized the seed bed with heat it is most disheartening to see those two tiny oval seedlings droop on their inch-high stems and die.

Marjoram, also, is very slow in germinating and the young plants are difficult to carry along until the warm nights come which are so much to their liking.

The delicate little annuals, anise, coriander, dill and a few others resent transplanting of their seedlings, and these must be carefully watched and covered on unusually cold nights after their transfer into the open.

But in this climate in order to give time to some of our woody perennial herbs, like lavender, sage and winter savory, to "set wood," if they are to withstand their first New England winter, we must sow their seed in flats or pots under cover by the first of March. With a few species fall sowing with fresh seed is successful. If the seed is very fine, the soil must be thoroughly soaked, pressed flat and hard, leaving as little air space as possible between the particles, and no standing water. Make very shallow drills with the edge of a ruler and sift the seed gently and thinly from the paper envelope into these depressions. Press firmly the whole flat at once with a board. Cover with the thinnest sifting of fine sand. If the flat is covered with a board or burlap and kept not too warm, there will be enough moisture until germination starts, unless the seeds germinate very slowly.

If the soil dries out, the flats or pots should be set in a tub of water to half their height. The water should soak up from underneath, for even a fine spray from a syringe sometimes dislodges and scatters the tender germinating seeds.

Convenience in handling is alone sufficient reason for using the small flats, not more than 12 by 10 inches.

If the climate is such that we may sow early in the open garden, many of our problems are solved. The seedlings are less likely to "damp off," and thinning takes the place of transplanting. As to the time of sowing, all depends upon the season and the warmth of the ground. By May 15, in Lexington (Massachusetts), I try to have all my seeds planted.

All sorts of superstitions once attended the sowing of seeds, but needless to say how important it is to order and plant fresh seed.

Who cares, nowadays, whether herbs are sown on the fulling of the moon and culled on the waning? We dare transplant parsley without fear, sow its seed on Good Friday and do not consider it necessary to steal our rue from a neighbor's garden to ensure its growth in our own. Even should we dare pull mandrake from the earth without the help of the historic chain and dog, and we have no feeling at all about the enmity which exists between basil and rue, and simply don't plant them together because rue likes chalky, poor soil, and basil likes good loam. Nor do we plant coriander, dill, and mallow together because "they love to grow near each other," but because grouped thus their feathery leaves and flowers make a harmonious color scheme.

Yet in the planting of elder at the corner of the herb garden do we way down deep remember the compassionate, protecting love this shrub has for all human beings? And aren't we a bit self-conscious as we leave our herb garden to its care, sure that its great white umbels will protect man and plant alike from all evil?

Sir Hugh Platt, Knight, 1659, bids us "Sow Coriander seeds in February, respecting the moon as in anise seeds." But let New Englanders heed him not, for I know coriander seed is best sown in the open ground in early April, whether the moon be in ascendency or not.

If seedlings have to be brought along in the house, they should have a sunny window without draughts and be in a room absolutely free from gas fumes. To harden them off, when the weather is warm, I transfer all boxes to a sunny piazza, often bringing them in at night. Of course to the owner of a greenhouse or frames this is all superfluous information, but most of us, after all, are window gardeners with small transplanting ground at our disposal.

All seedlings do need regular and *not* intermittent supervision. The herb beds should be made ready with the soil needed for each herb. Old plaster rubble is excellent to mix with the soil for the thymes, burnet and lavender, and rosemary. A fairly rich bed with compost and loam — *not* manure, which engenders rust — is needed for the mints, tarragon, lovage and angelica, although even these herbs like soil with a slight alkaline reaction. Some shade is needed for hyssop, the mints and woodruff; lots of sun for basil and chamomile and marjoram.

Transplant on a cloudy, windless day as late as possible, so that the seedlings may get the benefit of the night dew. It is surprising how much this helps establish the precious things in their new environment. Before the sun is too high the next morning I spread newspapers over the more tender herbs to hold the moisture around their roots.

Before transferring the seedlings from the flats to the seed grounds I water both flat and the open bed thoroughly. When the little plants are once in, there is less chance for air holes and subsequent drying of the tiny roots. The tufted, fibrous roots of thyme seedlings are ten times as long as the overhead plant itself, and recognizing this the gardener naturally makes a long, deep hole that the little plants may take root more quickly than they would if carelessly doubled up.

According to size of the mature plant, the distance between seedlings is gauged, and then only is some culling of weeds necessary until the growing plants cover the ground around. If mints are to be planted with other herbs, the spreading root stalks must be confined by a sunken galvanized border or by some other means, for they are great trespassers and voracious feeders. I planted a row under the trellis on one side of a grape arbor. It was very successful in the partial shade. Along the other side of the trellis, which was open and sunny, I planted parsley of all kinds. This made a lovely and harmless combination, for the thick parsley growth acted as a barrier, and sent the mint roots in another direction under the arbor.

I believe that some place in the home grounds may be found for any herb to grow; so no one need despair for lack of opportunity or space for an herb garden. At the same time all herbs respond gratefully to their individual needs of shade, sunlight, soil and moisture.

Lovage and angelica grow well near parsley; tarragon and balm like the same kind of soil. If mints and Roman wormwoods are planted in raised beds with deep paths between them and the paths are hoed constantly, I can keep their roots out of my thymes and marjorams. Outside of artificial barriers, that is the only way I know.

A rough bank around an old house, carelessly filled in with rubbish by contractors and too lightly loamed, makes an ideal green bank for thymes. Rosemary leans against the underpinning of the house for it likes the warmth of supporting walls. A few half-buried rocks keep the earth from washing off the slope. Also they make protected, sheltered little pockets in which to plant bulbous herbs like fritillaries, saffron and snowflakes (*Leucojum*) which come up through the fresh green of the thyme foliage.

As to winter covering, that, too, is wholly dependent upon the locality and climate where the herbs are growing. Snow is, of course, the ideal winter covering, but the thawing and freezing in a New England winter make January and February the zero hour for our lovely wintergreen herbs, about which an article was written in *Horticulture*, 1932. A soft thaw and frosts too often heave the plants out of the ground. If possible, press them back in the mud with hand or boot-toe. A smooth plank stays handy by the thyme beds and I ruthlessly lay it flat over the upheaved little plants and walk on it.

A covering of evergreen branches about Christmas time, when the ground is hard frozen, will save many a shrubby thyme. If piled around the santolinas, lavenders and germanders, but always leaving breathing space, these shrubs will have a better start in the spring. A light, natural covering of leaves will do the herbs no harm, though it is not always necessary.

Raising herbs from seed is not always practical, and the owner may find his garden best started with nursery-grown plants or from cuttings or root division. The proverbial friendliness among herb lovers never fails to provide plenty of material with which to start a garden. Today, an increasing number of nurseries will provide correctly named, pot-grown perennial herbs.

Even though there may be some repetition, the following lists may help the gardener whose interest in herb gardens is just beginning.

Ambrosia, sweet basil, sweet fennel, sweet marjoram, sweet mugwort, anise, borage, cumin, dill, German chamomile, false saffron, summer savory, pot marigold; these herbs are annuals, all easily grown from seed. They die, root and top, every year and need to be resown the following spring, or two plantings may be made in the same season. They may self sow, and such seedlings make much better plants than those from the first sowing.

Perennial herbs, which may best be propagated and increased by root division, layering or cuttings are perennial artemisias, costmary, horehound, hyssop, lavender, winter or wild marjoram, true mints, rosemary, rue, sage, southernwood, tansy, tarragon, thyme, wormwood, yarrow and some alliums. Beds of these herbs may persist for several years, although it is well to renew the plots at least every three years.

Fennel, if it does not winter-kill, should be included, not as an annual, but as a good perennial.

Make cuttings or slips of shrubby, woody herbs like

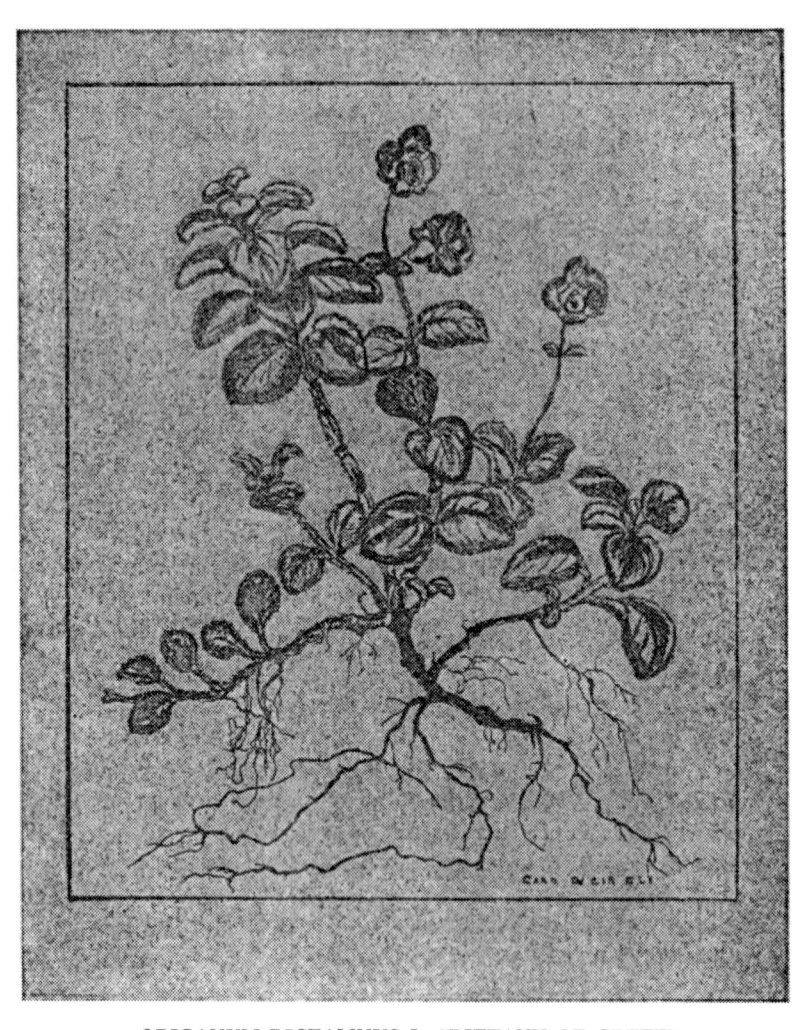

ORIGANUM DICTAMNUS L. "DITTANY OF CRETE"
Original etching by Caroline Weir Ely
This plant was propagated in Wenham, Massachusetts
from root brought from Crete in 1936

GENERAL HORTICULTURAL DIRECTIONS FOR HERB GARDENS 95

santolina, thymes, hyssops, rosemary and southernwood from new growth. Use sharp sand, thoroughly wet and packed.

Biennials, or the herbs which may have a life cycle of only two years, are caraway, clary, chervil, parsley, leeks. If the seed of these herbs is planted in late spring, by fall they should have formed good roots and tops that should carry the plants through the following winter. If biennials are sown in early spring they are likely to blossom early, set seed, and die. Often a true biennial may have its life lengthened by cutting all flowering stems. It is hard to say whether angelica shows the more frequently a biennial or a perennial history. Chervil is often treated as an annual.

Those herbs with more or less color, gray, green or bronze, are called "evergreen."* These persist through the larger part of a New England winter. Because of these characteristics they are valuable horticultural assets to the landscape architect. In the "Check List of Herbs for Modern Gardens" (see page 141), it is stated under *Thymus* which of the thymes are evergreen. However, if the ground is too wet, any thyme will winter-kill.

Until December, we may count upon the gray of santolina, lavender, horehound, sage, and several artemisias. Rue and southernwood sometimes begin to show new green tips as early as March. Burnet, hyssop and winter savory have more or less persistent green foliage. Wild marjoram makes a thick, soft, winter ground cover which seldom loses its green color. Lamium and the bugles have some evergreen varieties. Ground ivy is green the year round.

Also there is much to say about herbs as substitutes for grass and ground cover. Only very low-growing herbs, close clinging to the earth and which benefit by the lawnmower, will make satisfactory grass substitutes. Chamomile lawns are not made in this country as easily as in England where the moist climate keeps them thick and green the year round. Low herbs which have underground or creeping stems, make

---
*See *Horticulture*, May 1, 1932.

good ground covers. Not all ground covers are substitutes for grass.

Thymes are invaluable for the so-called "Alpine Lawn" and for the barren borders of roadsides on the public highways. Here the cost of grass maintenance is too often pro-

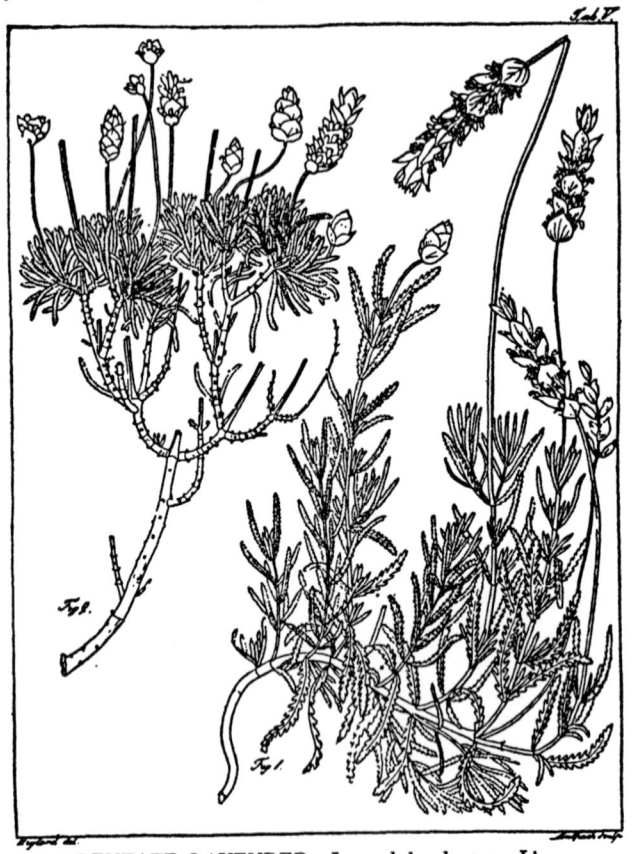

DENTATE LAVENDER—*Lavandula dentata* Linn.
*Fig. 1, var. vulgaris. Fig. 2, var. B. Balearica
From "Histoire Naturelles des Lavandes" de
Lassarez, 1826*
*Courtesy Publication Committee, Herb Society
of America*

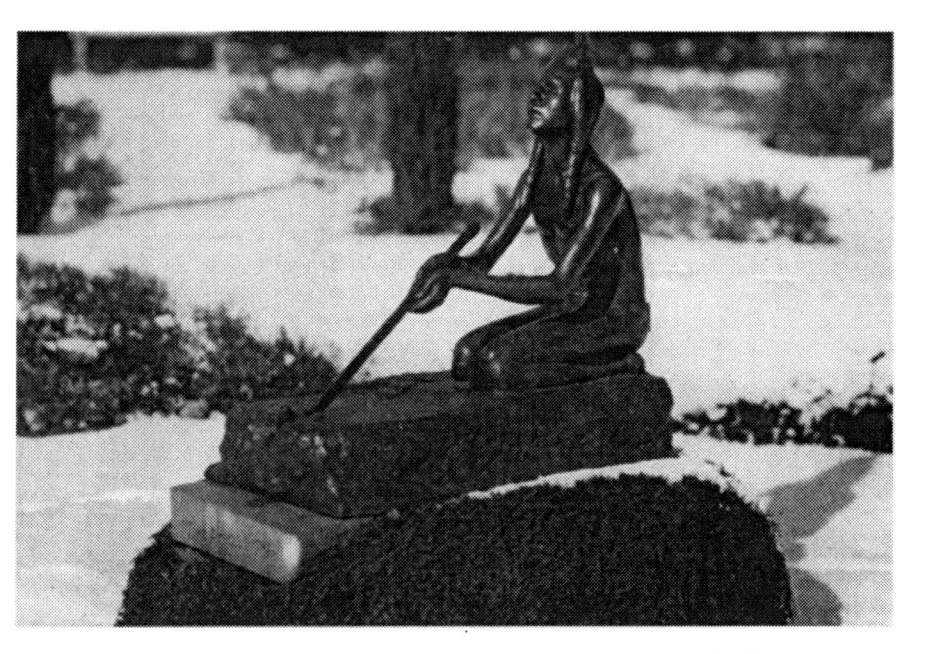

"TIME AMBLES WITHAL" Sundial in herb garden of Miss Annie B. Jennings, Fairfield, Conn. Note use of evergreen thyme on pedestal mound.

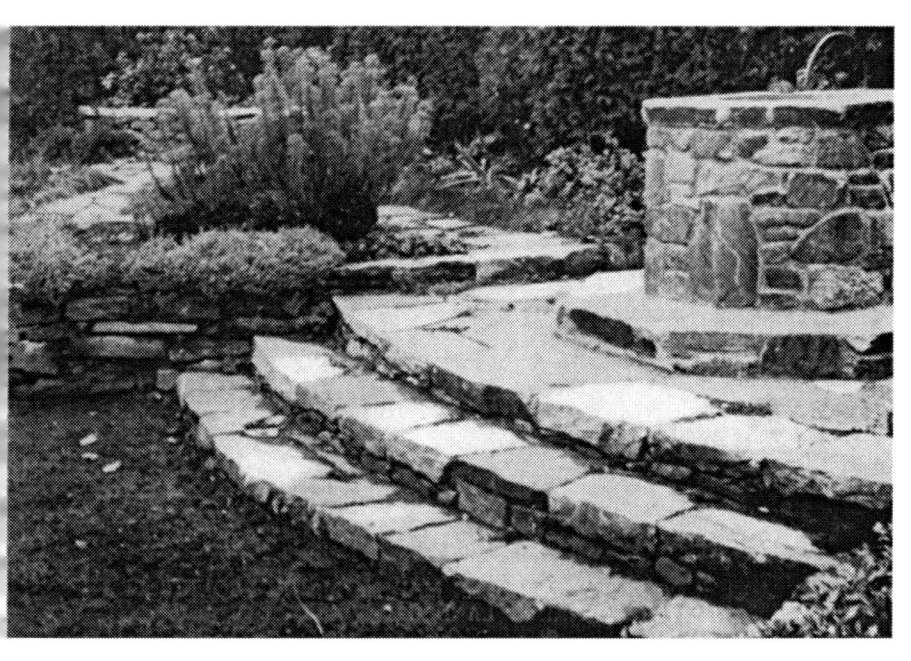

DIPPING WELL IN THE BEAUTIFULLY DESIGNED AND PLANTED HERB GARDEN of Dr. and Mrs. Maurice Ostheimer, "Grimmet," Whitford, Pa.

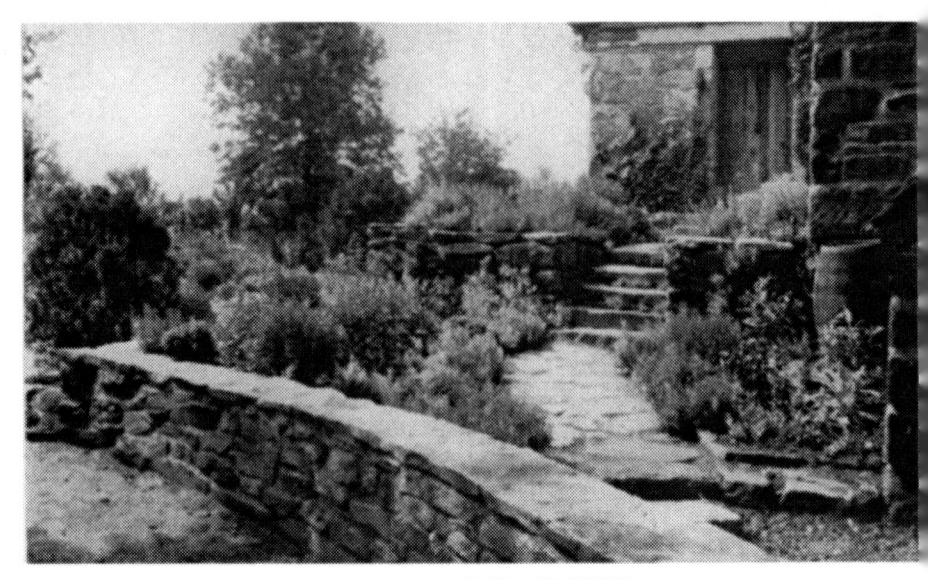

DOORSTEP PLANTING OF HERBS
Home of the late Mrs. G. C. F. Bratenahl, Weathered Oak Herb Farm, Bethesda, Md.

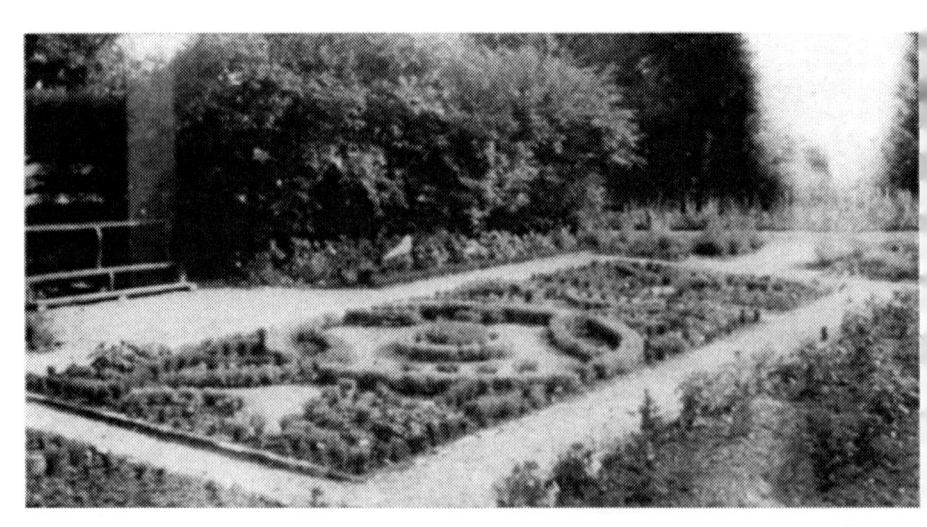

CULTIVATION OF HERBS HAS BEEN MADE A MAJOR PROJECT AT THE LOWTHROPE LANDSCAPE SCHOOL.

hibitive. But even were this not so, the herbs with their bloom and fragrance give unusual pleasure.

To take the place of grass I know of no better herb than *Thymus serpyllum Annie K. Hall,* which, in combination with the crimson and white thymes, is usefully resistant to winter-killing. Low ground-cover herbs are the bugles, dead nettles or *Lamium,* mountain thyme, and a number of other species. (See "Check List of Herbs for Modern Gardens," page 141.) Ground ivy, or as it is often called, Gill-over-the-ground, is best of all.

When Lord Bacon gave this advice in his essay "Of Gardens" in the last half of the sixteenth century, he anticipated one of the loveliest horticultural uses for herbs—that of ground covers.

"But those that perfume the air most delightfully, not passed by as the rest being Troden upon and Crushed, are three, that is Burnet, Wild Time, and Water Mints. Therefore, you are to set whole alleys of them to have the Pleasure when you walke or tread."

Taller, more shrubby herbs for moist places are lemon balm, peppermint, spearmint, costmary, bee balm, tall mugwort, woolly mint and the white strawberry.

Of not the least horticultural value are the low-growing compact herbs for filling in spaces between bricks or other pavings and edges of walks. The stones make cool root-runs for the plants, which usually grow well and, if carefully chosen, certain species will add a refreshing interest to the garden walk (see "Check List of Herbs for Modern Gardens," page 141).

Between the ascending wall boundary and the last row of paving stones a few taller but slender little herbs not over six or eight inches break a "set" line. English thyme, German chamomile, cobbler's bench and bugle might be thus used. They should look as though they had established themselves here from chance seeding.

No shrubby herb should be used in the walk itself nor one too tender to stand the tread of feet. Evergreen species are of course most desirable.

Of the *Thymus serpyllum* varieties, *T. albus, T. coccineus, T. Annie K. Hall, T. britannicus, T. lanuginosus,* and *T. pulchellus* are best for crevice planting.

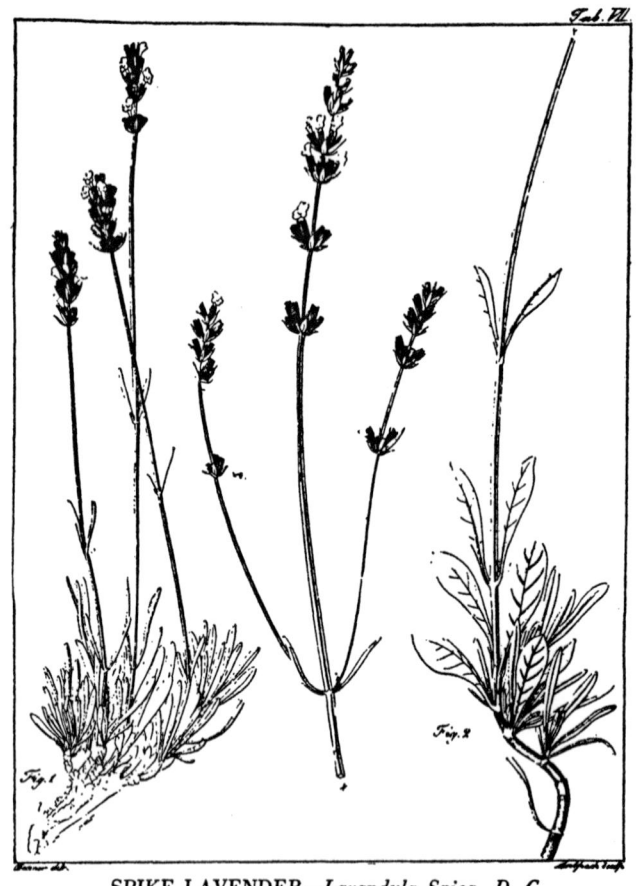

SPIKE LAVENDER—*Lavandula Spica,* D. C.
Fig. 1, *a vulgaris.* Fig. 2, *B. ramosa*
From "Histoire Naturelles des Lavandes" de
Lassarez, 1826
*Courtesy Publication Committee, Herb Society
of America*

A good combination planting is that of the crimson and woolly thymes. The gray of the latter species tones down the vivid magenta bloom of its companion which in turn serves as a winter protection for the more tender woolly thyme. Corsican mint, *Mentha requieni*, makes sweet-smelling mats between the stones, but it almost never lives through a cold winter. However, spring finds its seedlings everywhere.

Achillea tomentosa is a sturdy gray woolly little herb for broad cracks but its yellow flowers must be ruthlessly clipped.

Not all herbs used for borders are good edging herbs, which should, of course, be low, compact shrubs (see Knot Gardens, page 41). Taller herbs which may be used for outlining a larger garden should be kept clipped and bushy. Hyssop, especially the white variety, is a glossy green evergreen, ideal for this purpose. Other border herbs are rue, santolina, white sage (*Salvia officinalis alba*), rosemary, and box. For New England gardens a dainty edging infrequently seen is hedeoma, the wild pennyroyal, a soft-leaved, fragrant little bush.

There is much to say about the use of herbs for window gardens,* and there has been increasing interest in this phase of herb gardening. All herbs are by no means adaptable to the living room of a modern house. The atmosphere is too hot, too dry and airless. But if we understand their limitations and do not expect too much, there is real enjoyment in experimenting with the different groups for culinary or other household pleasure.

Of course the annuals whose life span is short at best, basil, coriander, anise, dill, fennel and borage, die soon after flowering.

Seedlings of these herbs should be potted in their containers in August, and left out-of-doors till well established. Glazed pottery makes the best container, for the roots do not

---

*See *Horticulture*, Feb. 15, 1933, "Sweet Herbs for Window Gardens."

dry out as quickly as in the common clay pot. For house plants they should be planted more closely.

The kitchen window box is fairly sure of success if the following directions are observed.

In early September, fill a small window box with good potting soil (three parts loam and well-rotted manure, a little bone meal and lime rubble or old plaster, one part sand, one part compost). Sow seeds of white mustard, garden cress, dill, basil and fennel. Cover the earth from the hot sun, keep in a cool, shady corner, bring into the house before freezing and use the aromatic green leaves for your salads and sandwiches as long as they last. Mustards and the cresses germinate very quickly within a day or two after sowing. They will even sprout like oats when sown on wet cotton in a saucer. But they do give us healthful greens and certainly can be grown by anyone who has a sunny window in which to place them.

If a kitchen window box of biennial or perennial herbs, parsley, chervil or mints is desired, take up young plants in late summer and make a separate box of the same good potting soil. Leave out of doors, protected by leaves from too early frost, until perhaps the last of September. Indoors, give them a cool window with some sun. The mistake too often is made of trying to grow parsley and chervil in too warm a room. They like far better a sunny shelf in a cold pantry.

Spearmint, peppermint and orange mint make good house plants, both charming and useful.

Among the few very interesting herbs which I have seen growing indoors is the Corsican mint, a clump of which was planted in a shallow milk pan, and kept in the sunny kitchen window of a farmhouse. It filled the pan full with fragrant tiny leaves and stems which were covered in February with infinitesimally small blossoms.

In a nearby farm was another herb growing in an unheated room, a hanging pot of the woolly thyme (*Thymus*

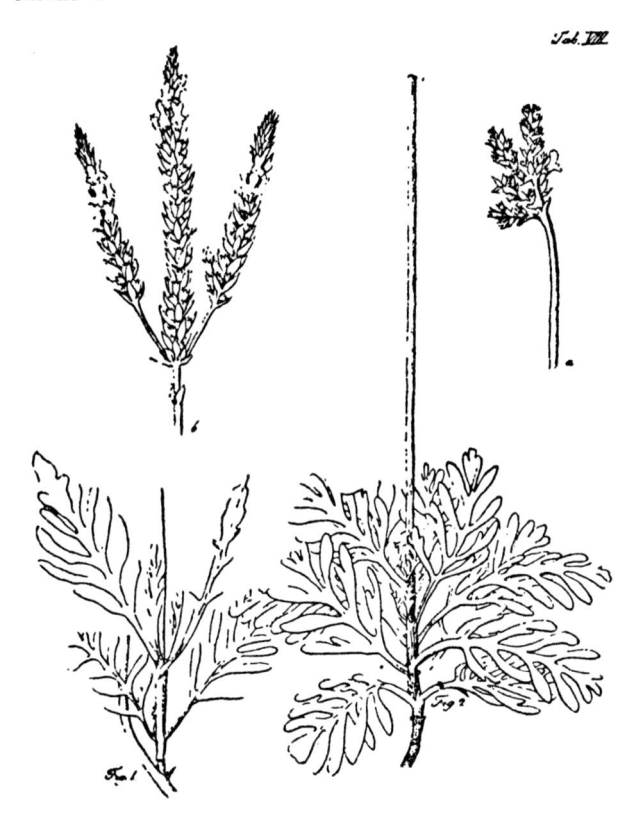

PINNATE LAVENDER—*Lavandula pinnata,* Linn.
Fig. 1, var. a. Fig. 2, var. b.
From *"Histoire Naturelles des Lavandes,"* de
Lassarez, 1826
Courtesy Publication Committee, Herb Society of America

lanuginosus). That atmosphere was much to its liking and its soft gray, lacy stems hung from the pot on all sides.

When growing indoors, sweet marjoram and santolina change their characteristic growth from stiff little shrubs to

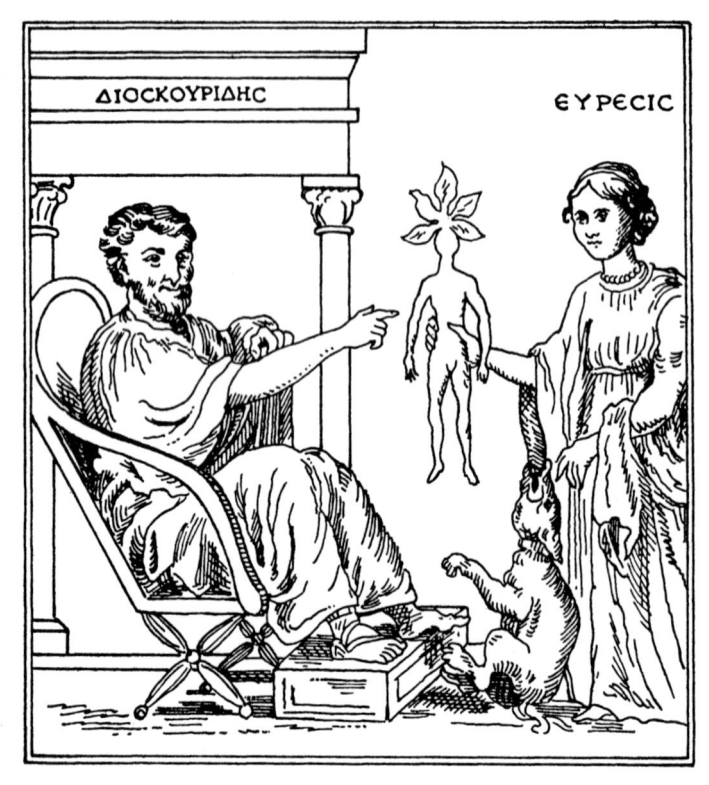

102   HERBS

Dioscorides receiving a root of the Mandrake from the Goddess of Discovery from Gunther's *Greek Herbal of Dioscorides*, 1934.

lax, trailing stems; but they are equally lovely. As to care of the herbs in the living room or kitchen, there is the usual treatment of watering regularly and keeping the plants free from plant lice. This can be accomplished by spraying, before bringing into the house, with a soapy solution and some nicotine insecticide. At intervals of about two or three weeks this should be repeated. Once in a while, plunge the whole plant, pot and all, into the tub. Give all sun possible and on warm days, fresh air.

These rules for window gardening with herbs may be applied to porch boxes and greenhouses.

Then of course there are the old favorites of the Victorian parlor window whose native home is in a far warmer country than New England—dittany of Crete and scented geraniums.

There are tender herbs which because of their exceeding fragrance and associations belong in the summer garden with other herbs. This list includes a few.

OLD ROSES and SCENTED GERANIUMS.

CEDRONELLA or MOSQUITO BUSH, *Agastache cana*

SUMMER LAVENDERS, see "Check List of Herbs for Modern Gardens," see page 158.

LEMON VERBENA, *Lippia citriodora*
ROSEMARY, *Rosmarinus officinalis*
TRUE MYRTLE, *Myrtis communis*
PINEAPPLE SAGE, *Salvia rutilans*
DITTANY, *Origanum dictamnus**

"Lavender and Rosemary! Two good old friends not to be cast aside for new comers. Treat them well, yet without grudge of shears in due season. Then, come summer—come winter,—green of Rosemary—gray of Lavender—will breathe out new lessons of stainless fragrance and steadfast faith to stir within us nobler thoughts than we sometimes harbor of the loyalty which wearies never though time steps on."—From "English Gardens," by Cook.

---

*See *The Herbarist*, 1936, Publication Herb Society of America, "Dittany Redivivus," Anne Burrage.

CHAPTER VIII

COMMERCIAL GROWING OF HERBS*

*Adapted from a letter from Mrs. E. B. Cole,
of Hamilton, Massachusetts
Director of Commercial Research in the Herb Society
of America*

The commercial growing of herbs for the wholesale market, whether for condiment, insecticide, or medicinal purposes, involves a different method of procedure from that of the cottage garden industry, and should be undertaken only by good growers, who, like farmers and market gardeners, have experience and equipment for acreage cultivation as well as the assurance of available labor.

In all cases, in addition to actual growing, knowledge must be acquired of the particular methods of harvesting and drying required to meet the specifications of the buyers of the particular herbs being grown. Special reapers for leafage, flower heads, or seeds are needed as well as specially constructed drying apparatus.

A crop grown for the seed market calls for different cultural treatment, and here enters the question of type, qualities, and better strains. A study of non-poisonous sprays and insecticides is imperative.

The commercial growing of medicinal herbs should not be undertaken even by experienced growers without first testing out soil conditions and climatic reactions in that section of the country where the project is undertaken.

As fairly little cultural information is as yet available, the grower of medicinals should have either close profes-

---

*"Notes on the Commercial Cultivation of Sage" and "1941 Records of a Group of Commercial Growers of Sage," Bulletins of the Herb Society of America by Sherman Hardy.

sional supervision or the background of experience to avoid the waste occasioned by failure. The value of this specialized crop is determined by the success with which the grower meets the specifications of the United States Pharmacopoeia, for on these requirements drug firms base their purchase of the crop. In many cases the potency of the herb must be determined by assays which are costly.

However, if the same scientific effort is used as that in developing other crops, commercial growing of herbs as a minor crop may become a profitable venture even after foreign imports again flood the market. A superior product means increased potency of the herb and higher yield. But there is need of carefully recorded experiments from different sections of the country as well as cooperation among growers to make their findings available.

CHAPTER IX

DRYING AND CURING HERBS

IT WAS after a talk with a group of garden lovers that a friend wrote me:

"Your lecture takes me back to my grandmother's 'corn chamber.' There were bins for beans and dried products of the farm; and the rafters were hung with braided seed corn and rows and rows of herbs.

"During the summer we children were allowed to have our dolls up there, and I can smell all the herbs now when I think of the happy hours I spent there as a child.

"I can remember how proud I was when my childish hands picked some Penny-ry-al and grandmother hung it up with the rest of the herbs. Well, all that is a blessed heritage!"

Throughout the summer conservation in the herb garden goes on apace. We use the fresh green leaves of parsley, chervil, the cresses, dill, lovage, angelica, thyme, sage, savory, marjoram, if happily for us they are at hand. Tarragon dried loses flavor. Horehound dried has less bitterness and should be so used. All seeds are more pleasantly aromatic when dried. The vile taste of coriander's fresh seeds is well known. Lemon balm and the true mints, peppermint and spearmint, as well as lavender and rosemary, are distilled commercially for their precious oils in spite of these days of synthetic products. But this process of distillation is not for an unskilled amateur, though a fascinating idea to play with. Dill, fennel and lovage leaves seem to me always to lose strength in drying. A drop or two of the pleasant dill oil answers all culinary purposes when that flavor is called for in the kitchen.

The herbaceous herbs, sweet marjoram and its kind, are cut for drying in their midsummer richness of growth just as they are ready to bloom. The whole plant, clean and dry, is cut.

A very good method to employ in drying parsley and celery tops, if in small quantities, is to dip the stem and leaves quickly into boiling salted water, shake them dry and spread on racks in a cool oven. When thoroughly dried they may be stored in tightly covered tin cans.

Horehound, thyme, sage, basil, savory, balm and marjoram are best dried slowly on racks in an airy room. Sunlight dissipates the aromatic oils in these leaves. When all moisture is out of the plants they should be crumbled, stems removed, and put in tins, not stored in paper. The less powdered the product the better and more lasting the flavor. If not completely dried before storing they will mould or there will be deterioration of their aromatic oil content.

Lavender flowers should be dried on their stems before the tips are in full bloom. Calendulas are dried before all the florets in the head are fully open.

The seeds of cumin, fennel, dill, coriander, caraway, bene and anise are used more often than the leaves and stems. The seeding heads should be cut on as short stems as possible as soon as ripe. Watch out for coriander: its seeds are heavy and big and drop to the ground almost as soon as they ripen.

Spread the seed crop for a week or so in a dustless, windless dry room on an old clean sheet. The attic chamber has its uses. Turn frequently, and finally, with gentle rubbing through the hands, the seeds are released from their stems, and the chaff is easily winnowed in a gentle breeze on a very dry day. Of course we are attempting no commercial threshing on a large scale in our small herb gardens, but to garner even an ounce is joyful triumph. The seeds must be clean and dry when you finally bottle them tightly, and you may be sure no produce that you buy will give you more epicurean flavor.

Drying out the roots of angelica, lovage, sweet flag, comfrey, sarsaparilla, ginseng, sassafras and other herbs is a slow process. Artificial heat is sometimes used. They are dug when growth has practically ceased in the fall and the storage of plant food materials in the cells is complete. However, I am told that sweet-flag root dug in the spring is more tender for "sugaring." Heavy roots like burdock are split and spread on wire trays. All dirt is carefully washed off and sometimes it is necessary to scrape the outside. The dried roots may be stored in heavy sacks, or paper flour bags, which are good containers. The roots are ready then to cut for candy, homemade beers and flavors.

At any rate, however crude our methods of salvage in the herb garden, nothing material or immaterial should be wasted. Every dried leaf and flower may go into the potpourri and cookery, that the whole herb garden may be conserved into the keenest aesthetic enjoyment.

To read of the industry of the Shaker brethren, when in their settlement at Harvard, Massachusetts, they built their great new Herb House in 1848, is to take a refreshing and soul-heartening glimpse into the simple, unaffected lives of those good men and women.

Read their journal of a year's work at Harvard, Massachusetts, for 1850:

"February 14, 1850: After meeting in the evening we got some help and put up 18 dozen large cans of Thyme till 12 o'clock."

"September 10, 1850: Cut the Hyssup and Sweet Balm."

"September 11, 1850: A company of brethren and sisters go to Chelmsford to pick Wintergreen."

"May 2, 1851: Set our Wormwood, Marshmallows, and Thyme roots," and May 2, "Transplant Horehound and Sage to the West Garden."

"Christmas day 1851: After the solemnities of the day are past, I paper a lot of herbs."

CHAPTER X

USES OF AN HERB GARDEN

WHOEVER possesses an herb garden today finds content and happiness the year round in the utilization of its simples. Our ancestors from time immemorial made from them their medicinal teas, tinctures, confections, syrups, salves, liniments and dyes.* They used the leaves for plasters and the flowers for perfumes and wines. They believed in and lived by the old Bible precept: "The grass grows for cattle, and herbs for the service of man and the leaf thereof shall be for medicine." †

Few parts of the sweet herbs failed of some use in nosegays or posies, scent bags or pomanders, and cookery of all sorts. After perusal of the many books on housewifery and cookery in the seventeenth and eighteenth centuries, it requires no flight of the imagination to picture the dilemma of a cook in those days bereft of her garden of sweet herbs.

Aside from their material uses, there is embedded in our very souls a faith in their mysterious magic. Who doubts the power of sweet marjoram to bring happiness to the spirit freed from the grave on which it grows, and the association of mugwort with the weary traveler? The cloister gardens furnished the flowering herbs for the church's most sacred festivals, and victors were crowned with their chaplets.

I do not like to think that there is an ancient use of sweet herbs not applicable today, but just where or how, in our modern civilization, we should revive that custom of "herbstrewing" I have been unable to conjecture. A friend

---

*See *The Herbarist*, 1936, Publication Herb Society of America, "Dyeing With Herbs," Frances T. Norton.

†See *The Herbarist*, 1938, Publication Herb Society of America, "The Empress Komyo," Harriet Addams Brown.

told me how, on a hot auto trip in the South, she trampled branches of mint on the car floor, bringing thereby cooling, wonderful refreshment to the atmosphere. In the luxury-filled days of Nero, mint, sweet calamus and saffron were strewn on the floors of Greek theatres and Roman baths. Later, rue, hyssop and meadowsweet covered filthy floors of mediæval castles and cottages. Sweet woodruff, lavender and rosemary made soft carpets in milady's bedchamber. In England rue, with its power over evil odors and vermin, was strewn in the judge's chamber even till the last century, which fact shows, in its long dying, the value of an old custom.*

John Parkinson, in his book, "A Garden of All Sorts of Pleasant Flowers," which he wrote in 1629, says: "There be some flowers that make a delicious Tussie Mussie or Nosegay both for Sight and Smell." Winter and summer, the scents of the herb garden were gathered into meaningful "posies," as the little old-fashioned nosegays were called. Alice Morse Earle renews our interest in a delightful chapter of her "Old-Time Gardens," and tells us that "a tussy-mussy was the most beloved of nosegays, and was often made of flowers mingled with sweet-scented leaves."

An old favorite of the fifteenth century was of marigold and heartsease — "of happiness in recollections" — though how marigold, which is our calendula, came by the meaning of grief ascribed to it in some old flower books is a mystery.

A red rosebud surrounded by forget-me-nots and southernwood signified devotion, undying memory and constancy.

The clove pink, or carnation, balm and hyssop told their story of resignation, pity and sacrifice; and if to them blue lavender flowers were added, the message included undying love.

"Mints were ever a good posie for students to smell of for it quickens the brain."

---

*See "Household Uses for Herbs" by Martha G. Stearns. Issued by the League of New Hampshire Arts and Crafts.

Red bee balm and southernwood with Bible leaf made the posie which, tucked into many a Sunday bodice, was sniffed to while away long hours of devotion.

Gray sage leaves and white and gold chamomile flowers symbolized long life, wisdom and patience.

A favorite valentine was the sprig of rosemary, sweet herb of remembrance, painted on a heart.

Sprays of rosemary tied into the bride's bouquet signified happiness which never failed.

The columbine was ever associated with folly, as was Jack-in-the-pulpit with zeal and ardor.

Gardener's garter is the old-time striped grass, which, escaping from civilization, was "always running back to green" and signified submission. This, with valerian, sweet rocket, and the sweet old semi-single peony, made another favorite nosegay.

Rue is perhaps the moly which Mercury gave to Ulysses, that he might better withstand the enchantment of Circe. Aside from its meaning of repentance, ascribed to it by Shakespeare and found nowhere else in the annals of plant lore or superstitions, it symbolized, to the ancients, clear vision and understanding.

Basil, in Italian folklore, means hatred, but curiously enough the Eastern countries endowed it with a meaning directly opposite. Violet's association is with death.

Balm was ever for sympathy and thyme for courage, sweetbriar's pink flowers for cheer, and burnet for a merry heart, with horehound's gray, wrinkled leaves for health.

A winter bouquet which must have given food for thought was made of bay for glory and yew for immortality, and holly for divination.

A decoction of periwinkle leaves administered to one's husband or lover recalls his erring devotion.

The soft, lacy leaves of gray wormwood were placed under the pillow in the hope that dreaming of it would bring domestic happiness, just as to dream of marigold augured for prosperity and a happy marriage. Heartsease and valley lilies surrounded by marjoram signified humility, purity and happiness.

Lavender blossoms bring luck to the wearer but primrose was associated with melancholy.

Alkanet, or anchusa, because from its roots was made the red dye which court ladies used in their lip salve, has since the earliest centuries been associated with falsehood, and this is its symbolism.

Foxglove stood for sincerity, fennel for flattery and broom for humility.

Mothering Sunday is May 15th, a day observed in England and set apart to revive an old custom when families met together in the home to bring gifts to the mother and worship together in the church of their faith.

Tradition of giving violets to the mother is enshrined in the old proverb, "Who goes a'mothering finds violets in the lane." — Taken from the *Guider*, England, March 1931.

The Christmas symbolism of the herbs is very lovely, and it is regrettable that it is not more often used.*

The Christmas creche becomes much more significant if in its making the folklore of herbs is used. Thyme made the bed of Mary. The little creeping pennyroyal was supposed to bloom at midnight, when the Christ Child was born, and it is said that Sicilian children place in the creche each Christmas a little pot of this herb.

Rosemary recalls the Presence in the garden, a memory of the Garden of Gethsemane with the quiet solitude of old olive trees under which the rosemary grew and blossomed.

Many of our herbs are green at Christmas time. The tiny gift nosegays are fragrant and delightful. A friend long ago added these lines to one she made for a friend:

> *"A sprig of Rosemary I give*
> *To speak of all the past—*
> *And Sage for life that's long and brave,*
> *With Balsam, sweet to last—*

*Here's Thyme to give you courage,
Mugwort to free from care,
Sweet Lavender a loyal heart—
That you may ever wear.*

*And on it all I gently lay
The Mistletoe for love
And may the little Christ Child send
His blessing from above."*

—NAN DANE

A nosegay for the blind is a "posie" of fragrant herbs. Southernwood, balm, mint, rosemary may awaken precious memories in those who cannot see.†

Well did our forbears know that Oriental proverb:

*"To raise flowers is a common thing
God alone gives them fragrance!"*

Connected with their symbolism, a book could be made of the superstitions of herbs and the special interpretations of herb dreams. From time untold, certain herbs have been dedicated to the evil one. There are herbs that the witches feared and used. There are herbs of divination and love. Far be it for a modern to say that there is no truth in the established traditions of centuries.

Yarrow, brought to the wedding, insured seven years' love. Violet was a proof against evil spirits.

To evoke the spirits the witches used mandrake, henbane, belladonna. Other witch herbs were dill, vervain, betony, mugwort and St. John's wort. The making of a witch garden, if cleverly constructed and planted, needs so truly literary research into the mediæval darkness of Anglo-Saxon superstition.

---

*See *Horticulture*, November 15, 1932, "A Wreath of Herbs and Evergreens."

†A useful and delightful little leaflet "What to Do With Herbs" by Margaret Norton is published by The Little House, Annisquam, Massachusetts.

There are so many ways, ancient and modern, for making potpourri and perfumes, flower scent bags and sachets that I am including merely a few suggestions to show this most æsthetic use of the herb gardens.*

The old recipes include often some commercial oil — bergamot, perhaps—salt, spices, and much manipulation. In the Still Room books of the seventeenth century are quaintly phrased rules for sweet waters and washing balls of scented herbs. Pomanders were made by sticking cloves as closely as possible through the skin of an apple, an orange, or a quince. Sometimes the ball was rolled in sweet orris powder. Bags of lemon verbena, rosemary and lavender flowers, according to Mrs. Earle, hung from the chair backs and bed posts just as we today use radiator bags filled with bayberry and sweetfern leaves. But I like to imagine that our colonists very early learned to mingle with their sweetness the resinous leaves of the fir balsam and the sweetgrass.

As I write, I am turning over in a little old basket a fragrant collection of dried leaves, petals and seeds, which, all last summer, I salvaged from house bouquets and the garden. To them no spice or salt has been added, and they have never been enclosed. I am trying to recognize all those sweet things which were tossed into that basket from time to time, and which dried out slowly and naturally without any artificial heat or sunlight. Perhaps the following suggestions may be helpful:

There are the pink petals of geranium and clove pink, the dried flowers and leaves of the sweet-scented varieties — skeleton-leaved, balm, rose, citron, nutmeg and peppermint geranium. Old-fashioned pink and white roses are here, also heliotrope, cowslip and valerian flowers. I recognize lemon-verbena leaves, the tips of santolina, balm, any number of thymes, marjoram and apple mint. There are costmary, sage, southernwood leaves, fragrant tips of sweet mugwort, dried sweet-woodruff leaves and blue violets.

*See *The Herbarist*, 1936, Publication Herb Society of America, "Herbs For My Lady's Toilet," Mrs. A. L. P. Dennis.

I have learned to guard against pennyroyal and other strong mints, like peppermint and spearmint, for their sturdy fragrance would overpower all others. But I love the dried flowers of lavender, the seed heads of bee balm, and a few yellow stigmas of saffron; also the hop-like, clustered fruits of the knotted marjoram which have a fragrance so different from that of its leaves. No one scent rises above the other, and the whole is blended into incomparable, lasting fragrance.

The blue flowers of bachelor's button and borage, and yellow calendula give color to the potpourri, though no added fragrance.

Gertrude Jekyll in "Home and Garden" devotes a grand chapter to the making of potpourri. That chapter is in itself a textbook on the subject.

A fragrant, efficacious rubbing lotion is made by putting sprigs of lavender leaves and flowers in alcohol and letting them stand, shaking occasionally.

Leaves of sweet basil and burnet steeped in boiling water make a cooling face wash.

Leaves of tall mugwort, *Artemesia vulgaris,* steeped in alcohol, make an excellent lotion for bruises.

Save the leaves of southernwood. Dry and powder for use in dispelling cooking odors. A pinch thrown on the stove or a hot pan or the open coals of a fireplace, wafts a most pleasing fragrance throughout the house.

A lover of Chinese gardens handed to me one day this poem, written 1144 B.C.:

>"*We load the sacrificial stands
>Of wood and earthen ware;
>The smell of burning southernwood
>Is heavy on the air.*
>
>*It was our father's sacrifice;
>It may be they were eased.
>We know no harm to come of it;
>It may be God is pleased.*"

Even today, how many old country cemeteries, both in the old and the new world, show none but fragrant, meaningful flowers planted on their graves!

Faggots of herb clippings saved from summer prunings should be kept, tied in bundles, and piled near the open fire. Then burn them when we need "the Mint's remembered fragrance."

Have you seen and smelled the lavender fans, which may call to mind the "nosegay nets" of the ancients? They are made by sewing pressed bunches of the flower stems into stiff nets cut fan shaped.

The roots of valerian make a perfumed powder called English orris and a medicine which is a powerful heart stimulant.

The exciting influence on cats is known to all who try to grow valerian in their herb gardens. Those animals roll in its leaves, bite at its flowers and revel in its intoxication. The legend is that the Pied Piper lured the rats from Hamelin with the valerian roots hidden in his shoes.

A strong decoction of the trailing stems and leaves and flowers of pennyroyal is a most efficacious and harmless wash for pussy's coat. I am assured that applications repeated every thirteen days will completely vanquish all fleas.

An Old Cough Remedy

A dear old lady made herself quite famous in her country corner of New England with this cough syrup, to the remedial qualities of which I attest. This is the rule as she gave it to me:

    1 ounce slippery elm bark
    1 " licorice root
    1 " boneset (thoroughwort)
    ½ " horehound

Break slippery elm and licorice roots into small bits and steep together with the boneset and horehound. Do not boil. After straining you should have about 3 half-pints of the liquid. Add 1 pint of molasses, and boil down until you have 3 half-pints in all.

A teaspoonful of this may be taken three or four times a day. One victim called this "a dark brown taste with bitter recollections," but it cured his cough!

Aromatic Vinegar

A very old Salem rule for mosquito bites has come to me from Mrs. Frances R. Williams of Winchester. She tells me that it was her grandmother's old rule; it might have been used for smelling salts and in the sick room.

1 ounce each of dill seed, lavender flowers, spearmint, rosemary, rue, sage and wormwood.

Add 1 gallon of cider vinegar, and let it stand in an earthen jar in a warm place, 5 days.

Strain and bottle, adding 1 teaspoon of pulverized camphor to each bottle. This will fill 5 wine bottles.

Snuffs

Snuffs were very important and several dried herbs were used in their preparation.

It is said, though some there are who deny it, that the quickening of learning in the early days of the Renaissance was due to the then recently-introduced custom of snuff-taking which revivified the senses and cleared the brain for thinking deeply. Betony made grand snuff, as did also the dry powdered leaves of lavender, sage, rosemary and asarabacca, marjoram and basil.

The dried leaves of basil taken as snuff were considered a cure for nervous headaches.

CHAPTER XI

HERBS AS A COTTAGE INDUSTRY

WITH increasing interest in herbs, small and sometimes profitable cottage industries have arisen in connection with small home gardens throughout the country. In order to encourage this activity, to furnish reliable information and also to eliminate disappointment in these ventures as well as financial loss, the Herb Society of America offers help to the herb gardener by publication of several timely bulletins.

The society defines cottage industry as the preparation of fresh home-grown products for retail sale. This preparation includes the growing, harvesting, blending and packaging of these fresh herbs for retail sale by the individual growers.

"It is not sufficient," they warn the seller, "to put on the market a unique container regardless of the quality of its contents." Blending different herb flavors is an art of a good cook, but of no avail if the herbs she uses are not carefully harvested and dried. Buyers are quick to discern and seek the best.

Selling fresh herbs from a well ordered and attractive roadside stand in connection with the farm home offers possibilities to the clever housewife, particularly if her locality is in a summer colony lacking home gardens. There are few shoppers who do not appreciate, in these vitamin-conscious days, a bowl of clean fresh salad herbs, and the more so if the herb garden from which they came is on view near by. More unusual herbs, not so often found in the open market, arouse curiosity which a few trials make a habit. Among them are young mustard leaves, tender, thin, curly lettuces where the whole plant is cut neatly from the root, sorrel, leeks and shallots, chives and a few leafy tips of fennel and tarragon.

Dill is in demand at pickling time when many a housewife is obliged to go far afield for this herb, as well as for fresh sage at Thanksgiving. I have seen a basket of basil seedlings sold with young tomato plants, and the fresh basil in canning time with a peck of ripe tomatoes; also a bunch of lemon thyme to cook with canning peaches and a carton of pot herbs accompanied by a bouquet of sweet flavoring herbs to add to the soup kettle. These small condiment nosegays, a few sprigs of thyme, and sweet marjoram with summer savory and a sheaf of chives bound round the stems, should sell well. Of course education of the buying public is sometimes a slow process but hard work, ingenuity and honest endeavor to give the purchaser herb products of only the highest grade should make this sort of cottage industry a success.

Pottery jars of horehound candy made with lemon thyme and no synthetic oil are always salable. Canned sorrel and tomato soup with a bouquet of the herbs used in their making might be shown near by. A bunch of rue, hyssop and burnet in right proportions suggests an improvement on canned cranberry cocktail. Charming little nosegays sell at fairs as fast as clever fingers can put them together.

If a small greenhouse is possible for housing the tender plants, tarragon and mint, properly forced, will yield fresh green leaves until spring, and there will be many a call for sweet and garnish herbs all winter, particularly when the Christmas festival calls for their sweet symbolism.

CHAPTER XII

COOKING WITH HERBS*

"In pottage without herbs there is neither goodness nor nourishment."

THE *cooking* or *culinary* herbs are used for flavoring soups, salads, stews, meat stuffings, bread foods and confections. They add piquancy to hot teas and cooling drinks.

Since the small home vegetable garden is usually a limited family affair, it is obvious that, as with vegetables planted, the herbs to be grown among them will vary likewise.

Which herb is most used in herb cookery is a question of the cook's individual preference.

If only ten strictly culinary herbs were to be chosen in order of preference, they might be parsley, sage, thyme, mints, marjoram, savory, chives, basil, tarragon, dill.

But when the French chef is deprived of chervil and lovage, the German of caraway and anise, the Oriental cook of cumin, coriander and sesame, cooking becomes to them a commonplace occupation.

In whatever form you use the herbs for seasoning, in herb cookery there is one unalterable rule. Never overpower with herb flavor the real taste of the viand you are seasoning.

A friend who is most successful and understanding in her use of herbs often warns those who seek her advice, "Use a light hand," she says, "You do not ask me how much salt or pepper to sprinkle on your foods!"

In cooking, herbs may be used dried or fresh according to convenience, but there is no question about the superiority of the fresh green sprays gathered from our own gardens.

---

*The reader will find invaluable "The Book of Herb Cookery" by Irene Botsford Hoffmann. Houghton, Mifflin Co.

Perhaps in time we shall make more use of the distilled oils of herbs. Dill oil certainly gives to potato salad a flavor equal to the fresh herb, whereas the dried leaves of dill have none at all. All success to the herb-minded chemist who is now experimenting with the distillation of the essential oils of burnet and tarragon.

Rue for its curious tonic flavor is regaining today its lost popularity, but it must be used most cautiously and only with foods harmonious to its bitterness, as in the cranberry cocktail, and in cream cheese sandwich filling with rye bread.

Rosemary is a taste, distinctive, and it is no modern notion to use the aroma of its leaves in bread and with boiled meats.

Sweet cicely and rose-geranium leaves laid on the bottom of the cake pan before pouring in the batter are survivals of its use thus a hundred years ago. The aroma of the baked cake is a mingled sensation of smell and taste, most appetizing.

Hyssop is an herb for which the cook of an earlier day had more use. Strong preservative herbs were useful in keeping meats and also in disguising their spoilage.

But like rue, hyssop's medicinal tang occasionally finds favor. I always shall feel indebted to the friend who told me to add a tip of southernwood to beet soup or "borsch." The flavor is indefinable, but there.

Thyme's flavor is so closely akin to its fragrance that the nose might be the guide when it is used for the bland vegetable soups with the pot herbs, parsley, sorrel and lettuce.

The potency of different species and varieties of basil gives opportunity for much argument among cooks, but all are indispensable in tomato cookery. They taste and smell like cloves which careful blending with other herbs can accentuate.

When to the cucumber flavor of burnet's leaves are added, the onion flavor of chives and the piquancy of parsley, particularly if the grated root of the turnip-rooted variety is used, each herb brings out the flavor of the other. If freshly chopped chive is sprinkled over the opened hot baked potato into which parsley butter has been folded, the effect is stimulating to the jaded appetite.

Of course the wild herbs contribute their quota of aromatic barks, roots, seeds and present added possibilities to the house wife in her search for delicate and snappy herb seasonings. Among them are sassafras whose dried leaves powdered make the soup-thickening file powder, sarsaparilla root, wild sweet cicely root and many others.

That this art of blending herb flavors has authoritative background is evidenced by numerous suggestions in old cook books of America and the earlier still-room books of England. Mrs. Leyel, when she writes about tansy, quotes Boerhaave, the Danish physician of the 16th century, "This balsamic plant (tansy) will supply the place of cinnamon and nutmeg." A slight cinnamon flavor is found in the dried and grated roots of elecampane, but add a fennel seed or two and imagination may not have to carry the cook quite so far. Thoughtful experimentation with our herb flavors will help the homemaker to surmount more cheerfully the trials of a depleted spice box.

As a people we have grown lazily dependent upon the herb-spiced processed meats of the great packing concerns. Conveniently canned foods of every sort have assumed an importance undreamed of even a decade ago. Now comes scarcity of tin, labor and spice, and present-day economic conditions bid fair to send the housewife back to all manner of home canning and food preservation and to her herb garden for spicing and flavoring.

In canning pork for sausage meat, spice with sage, marjoram, and thyme and a bit of savory for pepper. In canning fowl, add a small leaf of common bayberry. This is the leaf used by our early colonists who found its flavor not unlike the laurus leaf, or "bay," that they knew in their homeland. Home-canned stock of veal or beef is seasoned as in the trade with thyme, marjoram, and savory. Basil added, fresh or dried, to canned "mock turtle" soup removes it from the commonplace.

As for dill it is an herb with its own characteristic flavor. The seeds have a curious sweet bitterness comparable to no tropical spice. If its young tips are packed down between layers of salt in a crock we may enjoy its fresh green flavor on shell fish all winter.

A slight cucumber flavor is in the young leaves of borage, burnet and syringa (mock orange).

Sweet cicely, chervil, anise, fennel, lovage and giant hyssop (*Agastache*) give a decided flavor of licorice.

For peppery herbs use savory, costmary, basil and cresses.

To give a piquant, unusual taste in cake frostings, sweets and cookies, use dried coriander seeds, also caraway, cumin and sesame seeds; also flowers of saffron and marigold. Stems of angelica are candied; also the roots of lovage and sweet flag.

Anise, horehound and peppermint are the "candy herbs."

Dill, marjoram, savorv, mint have a place of their own in the dietary, for as carminatives they are either cooked with or sprinkled over starchy or otherwise hearty vegetables.

Sage, thyme, marjoram, parsley adapt their flavors to meat cookery, and basil, dill and fennel to fish.

It is true that these condiment herbs which have been used for centuries, add no calories to the dietary, and that they have no direct food value. Their part in the family menu is to bring savor to bland and tasteless foods, digestive piquancy to starchy vegetables and generally to relieve the flatness of routine cooking.

Herbs for liqueurs are the mugworts, peppermint, lemon balm.

To wines and fruit drinks or punches, lemon thyme, sweet woodruff, borage and the stimulating mints give interesting zest.

Among the "tea herbs" are peppermint, lemon balm, chamomile, lavender, spearmint, lemon thyme, sage, verbena and catnip.[*]

---

[*]See "Tea Herbs in Early America," by Helen Noyes Webster, *Herbarist* for 1940.

In 1770 there were in our Colonies "herb tea" and "store tea." Dried leaves, bark, roots or flowers of at least fifty herbs and shrubs or trees made hot, aromatic drinks for the patriots.

Later, as penetration into the American wilderness cut off the source of home supplies, the pioneers made much use of these stimulating and medicinal plants, and even today the mountain people know and use them.

Rose hip tea as well as jams, sweets, and sauces are made by stewing the fleshy red fruits of wild roses. Sweet homemade wine is sometimes added.

The Ojibway Indians made a cooling drink by stewing sumac berries in water with maple syrup.

A modern herbalist speaks derisively of the expensive cup of chamomile tea which, sweetened with sugar and cream, is served today in some exclusive New York beauty parlors, and suggests that its use is not different from that tea brewed to soothe the nerves of court beauties in the Middle Ages. To make it, first grow good German chamomile in your own garden. Cull and dry the flower heads as they come into bloom. Pour one quart boiling water on less than half an ounce of dried chamomile flowers. Let stand fifteen minutes, strain, sweeten with honey or sugar, and take at bedtime as a sure preventive of nightmare and for quiet sleep.

Wormwood, pennyroyal, catnip, sage, lavender flowers, fennel and mint teas are esteemed for their medicinal and tonic virtues. They are brewed, as is chamomile, and never allowed to boil. Crockery or enamel vessels must be used, for the acidity of the herbs discolors iron and tin and also taints the freshness of the brew.

A pharmacist once told me that if herbal brews and stewing fruits were removed from the heat "as soon as the aroma filled the room," no sweet essence was lost.

In summer lemon thyme, peppermint, verbena or pineapple mint enhance the flavor of "store tea." Place a green sprig in the cup and pour in the hot tea.

Combined with green China teas, an equal weight of dried Mitcham peppermint leaves and a few lavender flowers will make a drink as tonic as maté, which is made of the leaves of a tropical holly.

For punch and other cooling drinks* use iced tea, grape juice, raspberry vinegar, ginger ale, orange or lemonade as a base. For sweetening, honey is ideal with herbs. Even a small amount added to a boiled sugar syrup makes a "smoother" drink. Boil unpeeled sliced lemon or orange with the sugar and water in making the syrup. To this add lemon thyme, as much as you like, mints, or lemon balm. Strain, or, if the syrup is bottled for future use, leave in the herbs.

Spearmint is the best julep herb and is used without crushing.

The stimulating flavor of borage tips and flowers has always been recognized in claret drinks.

Sweet woodruff gives "snap" to champagne and white wine.

Always use clean herbs free from water in these beverages. Remember that the tips of young shoots are most pungent.

That wine or vinegar has ever been a favorite medium in which to preserve the aromas of sweet and savory herbs is recognized in the very earliest cook books. But it is with a good bit of Epicurean delight that we are today trying out these quaint old rules in modern kitchens.

Tarragon, basil, burnet lose much of their aromatic oil content in the drying process, but the aroma is well preserved in vinegar. In times far gone by, vinegars were also aromatized with rose petals, gilly flowers or clove pink, elder, rosemary and other spicy, scented blooms.

These flower vinegars redeem the most uninteresting salad and sauce and until we have used them we cannot realize how utterly prosaic is plain "store vinegar." Use good cider vinegar or white wine vinegar as a basis for something especially choice. It is a happy pastime if you take the container with you to the herb patch and pack the jar full of the succulent tips and leaves as fast as you pick. Press them down

---

*See "Olden-time Beverages," edited by Alice Earle Hyde.

hard in the vinegar, stopper and allow to stand on the sunny shelf a week or more. Then strain and add to the liquid more fresh herbs if you like, but I generally leave the jar as it is and use the vinegar-soaked leaves chopped in salad dressing the winter through. Of course the whole process is begun on a warm summer morning in July when the herbs are "juicy" with vigorous growth.

A mixed herb vinegar is useful, and the herbs which might be used are lemon balm, marjoram, thyme, basil, tarragon, chive, savory, burnet and a bit of rue. Here use discretion and let no one strong herb overpower another. Herbs most frequently used alone are basil, tarragon, burnet and mint.

Mint vinegar may also be made in another way, as follows: Bring to a boil one quart of unadulterated cider vinegar. Add one cup of granulated sugar, a pint of spearmint leaves and young stem tips. Stir and crush. Boil for a few minutes. Strain and bottle hot in glass jars. This is one of the best flavors for iced tea and fruit punches where fresh mint leaves are not at hand. It is also used as the basis of mint sauce for lamb and mutton cookery.

"The Cook's Oracle," revision, published 1823, reminds us that "the flavor of Burnet leaves resembles a cucumber so exactly that, when infused in vinegar, the nicest palate would pronounce it to be cucumber."

"Basil vinegar," the "Oracle" goes on to say, is "A secret the makers of mock turtle soup may thank us for telling—a tablespoon of this put in when the soup is finished will impregnate a tureen of soup with Basil and acid flavors at very small cost, when fresh basil and lemons are extravagantly dear."

While these herb vinegars are perhaps not a vitally important part of our food preservation program, they at least add zest to the vitamin-filled salad and replace to some extent imported spice aromatics.

Cordials to serve as aperitifs in the tiniest of glasses can be made from the herb garden in the home kitchen. Exact proportions depend upon the strength of the spirit used and personal liking of the herbs which flavor it. Briefly cordials are made by infusing young leaves and new tips of the herbs in brandy or alcohol. It may take several weeks before the desired strength is reached. The liquid should be strained through fine cheesecloth or other filter. A syrup is then added. This is made with sugar or mild-flavored honey and water. Alcohol is used for peppermint cordial, and brandy for tarragon. Wormwood (*artemisia absinthium*) with brandy makes what is known as bitters.

The three old "Stirrup Cup Herbs of Merrie England," hyssop, rue and burnet, find again a place in modern cocktails, though far be it from me to assert that their vitamin content is thereby increased.

Herb Punch

Pour three cups of hot orange pekoe tea over the leaves from a large bunch of mint, the same quantity of lemon balm and borage. Add the juice of nine oranges and six lemons and a syrup made of two cups of hot water and one of sugar. Let this steep for two hours. Then pour over a large piece of ice in a punch bowl. Add two quarts of ginger ale and one quart of white rock. Sprinkle blue borage flowers on top.

This rule was given me by Miss Ruth Gilmore and the punch is most delicious.

Tomato Cocktail

One peck of unpeeled tomatoes, a generous handful of celery, parsley leaves, 3 sweet peppers, onions to taste. Wash, stew all together, and rub the tomatoes through a strainer. Make from your fresh herbs a "bouquet" of basil, thyme, marjoram and savory, one sprig of each.

Bring the strained tomato liquid to a boil, add the herbs, with pepper and salt to taste. Strain through a coarse sieve, and bottle.

Serve very cold with a dash of lemon if desired, also garlic and celery or Worcestershire sauce.

Cranberry Cocktail

One quart cranberries, 1 pint sugar, 2 quarts boiling water. Boil till berries are soft, rub through a strainer, and add to the liquid a fresh "bouquet" of lemon balm, lemon thyme, burnet, hyssop and rue—a few sprigs of the first three but only one of rue and hyssop. Boil gently for 5 minutes, strain and bottle. This is equally delicious served hot or cold, and the herbs certainly do give a strength of character to the juice which is sadly lacking in the commercial canning of this popular beverage. Mint leaves, alone, give excellent flavor, but use the more delicate English apple mint or curly mint.

The importance of green herbs in salads* is stressed by the modern nutritionist. That salad making is no new art we realize when we read Cowper's translation of that great poem by Virgil, "The Salad":

> *"There, at no cost, on onions rank and red,*
> *Or the curled endive's bitter leaf, he fed."*

One of the first green salads with which I became acquainted was made with very young dandelion leaves and nasturtium flowers with half-open buds and tiny succulent leaves. Sorrel, chives and highland cress were used. The dressing was made of oil, lemon, vinegar with chopped thyme, chervil, tarragon, burnet and lovage. Leaves and dressing were mixed without crushing an herb or leaf.

For the usual green salad of endive, lettuce, chicory use this herb-and-honey dressing which Mrs. Bratenahl first suggested to me.

Dissolve ¼ cake of comb honey in juice of 1 lemon. Combine with 1 cup of salad oil and herb or flower vinegar (2 tablespoons). Add paprika and salt to taste and a pinch of celery seed.

Beat or shake till well mixed and add cut-up leaves of chives, tarragon, lovage, burnet, sorrel and perennial onion leaves which have been cut crosswise, so that they make little thin circles.

This should be a sweet dressing so thick with herbs that it must be ladled, not poured. It is most delicious blended thoroughly with the green salad leaves. Rub salad bowl with garlic.

Macaroni and Herb Salad

Boil elbow macaroni 20 minutes. Blanch quickly and cool. Don't let the pieces "glue" together. Chop garden thyme, burnet, savory, chives, tarragon, sorrel, a few leaves of each. Mix lightly with the macaroni. Sweet red peppers and stuffed olives may be added. Mix all with mayonnaise which has been slightly thinned with herb vinegar. Mound and chill. In serving, surround with halves of stuffed eggs, or the eggs may be hard boiled, chilled and cut into the macaroni. Stuffing for the eggs is made by mashing the hard-boiled yolks with lemon juice, salt, paprika and finely chopped parsley and chervil; mayonnaise if desired.

This sounds like a lot of work, but it's really easy with the garden close by and in itself this salad makes a well-balanced meal.

Soups and Meat Dishes

It is not always convenient to have ready in just the right proportion those very necessary combinations of flavorings for soups, but the "bouquets" may be prepared and kept ready for use.

Small cheesecloth bags about two inches square are filled with the special "bouquets" of *dried* herbs, labeled, and stored in tight tin containers.

The quantity given in the following recipes will fill three bags and in each is enough seasoning for about two quarts of liquid. The bags are dropped in the boiling soup toward the end of the cooking, and should be left in the kettle an hour or less according to taste. Long cooking makes herbs

---

*The salad lover will find pleasure and instruction in Evelyn's "Acetaria" (reprinted from its first edition of 1699 by the Woman's Committee of the Brooklyn Botanic Garden) and also in Cowper's translation of "The Salad," 1799.

bitter and destroys the fine essence of distinction between the different kinds in the "bouquet." The little sac of herbs should not be used again, though it often is.

Kitchen Bouquet for Consomme*

Two teaspoons dried parsley leaves; 2 teaspoons dried celery leaves (grated root of this herb may be used in place of leaves); 1 teaspoon each of garden thyme and sweet marjoram; ¼ teaspoon sage; ½ teaspoon savory; 2 large bay leaves crumbled; (if the true bay, *Laurus,* is not available, use leaves of wild bayberry, *Myrica).* Put 1 clove in each bag. (Use sage only when stock is made with pork or poultry.)

"Bouquet" for Fish Stock

Two tablespoonfuls crumbled celery and parsley leaves; ½ teaspoon each sage and savory; 1 teaspoon basil; ½ teaspoon fennel seed; 2 bay leaves, crumbled; 3 peppercorns; 3 cloves, 1 in each bag.

"Bouquet" for Tomato Soup

One small bay leaf; 3 peppercorns; 3 cloves (1 in each bag); ½ teaspoon thyme; 1 teaspoon basil; 2 tablespoons celery; and 2 tablespoons parsley.

"Herb Bunch" Soup

The faggots of fresh herbs used in this famous soup are always sold in Southern markets, but we may make them at home from our own herb gardens.

Three sprigs of parsley; 2 each of savory, sweet marjoram, and thyme; a stalk of celery with the leaves. Tie the bunch together with a leek, winding its leaves around the stems of the herbs.

To make the soup, follow any rule for making a rich beef broth with marrow bone and meat. Boil with onion, carrot,

---

*See "Blend Chart of Culinary Herbs in Common Usage" by Sherman K. and Vera B. Hardy. *Herbarist* for 1942.

cabbage, or any desired vegetable. Strain, cool, and remove fat. The faggot of herbs may be used in this soup before straining. To give a more pronounced herb flavor, however, boil them in the clear broth and remove before serving. This is a delicious "vitamin soup," piquant as a cold soup jelly for jaded appetites on a hot day.

Parsley, Sorrel or Lettuce Soup (Basic Rule)

Fry leaves of the pot herb in butter, stirring until thoroughly cooked but not brown; add flour and hot milk to the soup consistency desired, season with salt, paprika, and onion juice, rub through a sieve, reheat, and sprinkle on each serving chopped parsley leaves or chervil, or marigold flowers.

It is interesting always for the herb gardener to experiment with the blending of herb flavors, either from green herbs or from well-blended herb powders. Often the use of dried and powdered lemon or orange peel, with bay salt, will create some individual or unusually savory blend.

Roast Ham With Herbs

Parboil ham if necessary, dry, remove tough brown skin; rub with a paste made of brown sugar, fine crumbs or powdered cornflakes, into which are thoroughly sifted and mixed a pinch of savory, two pinches of marjoram, one pinch of basil and one pinch of thyme. Stick with whole cloves if you can get them or if not add more sweet basil. When all is ready for the oven, dip green sprigs of garden thyme and sweet marjoram in mixed herb vinegar and lay them over the roast. Pour a little herb vinegar into the pan, and as the ham browns, baste generously with the liquid. Cover and cook slowly.

For an Easter salad to serve with this roast, stuff halves of eggs with chopped mustard leaves, plenty of chives, a few tarragon leaves, and, of course, salt, lemon and paprika. Use chicory or young dandelion leaves for the "greens."

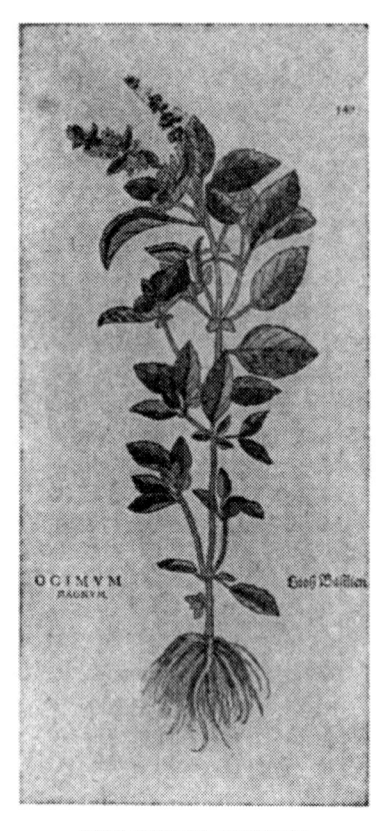

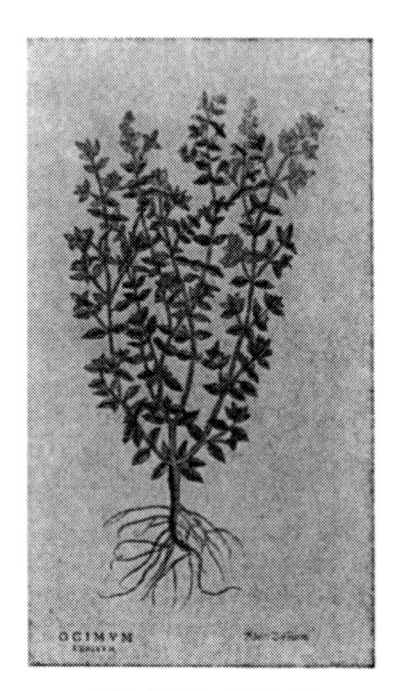

THE GREAT OCIMUM
SWEET BASIL

THE SMALL OCIMUM
BUSH BASIL

Taken from Latin Herbal *De Historia stirpium* (History of Plants) Written in 1542 by one of the most celebrated German Physicians Leonhart Fuchs.

Chicken With Herbs

Make a cream sauce with flour, butter and chicken fat. (If the fat is taken from stock in which onion, parsley, and celeriac, or the green leaves of celery have been cooked it is much more flavorsome.) Add ¾ cup of milk, ¾ cup of chicken stock, ½ teaspoon of salt with paprika or pimento to taste. Then add ½ teaspoon each of burnet and rosemary, 1 teaspoon each of chives, chervil, and tarragon, ⅛ teaspoon each of rosemary and garden thyme, and 1 cup of cut-up celery. (All herbs should be finely chopped.) Mushrooms may take the place of burnet and rosemary. Let all stand in a double boiler for half an hour or more. Serve the dish with herb buiscuit. If you have not all the herbs in your garden experiment with those you have. It is really lots of fun. Try it and see for yourself.

Carrots with lemon juice and mint go well with this chicken dish. Cook as follows: Melt a generous piece of butter, add the juice of 1 lemon and ½ tablespoon of chopped spearmint. Combine with 1½ cups of diced cooked carrots.

Served in the old Buckman Tavern, Lexington, Mass., by MRS. WILLIAM BALLARD, at a Garden Club Luncheon.

Omelet With Herbs

Everyone who has tasted this most delectable breakfast dish in Italy or France must realize how frequently egg dishes in this country are utterly prosaic.

The herbs for omelets may be gathered, chopped and kept fresh for some time in a closed glass jar in the refrigerator. Thyme, parsley, tarragon, chives and marjoram make the usual "faggot," or bouquet, and a bit of sweet chervil.

One tablespoon of milk to each egg used, salt and pepper to taste, a half teaspoon of butter for each egg, melted in an iron frying pan.

Beat whites and yolks together until light, add hot milk, and chopped herbs to taste. Turn into the melted butter, brown and fold, garnish with parsley or chervil leaves. If desired, a light, fluffy omelet is achieved by beating the yolks and whites separately, combining with milk, and adding chopped herbs just before folding.

Spaghetti-and-Tomato Recipe of an Old Roman Cook

Boil 1 pound of spaghetti 20 minutes. Drain dry. Toss into a frying pan of hot oil (1 cup) in which has been previously browned 1 chopped onion, or 1 clove of garlic and a few leaves of sweet basil, green or dried.

Turn the spaghetti constantly with two forks, lifting it until the whole is thoroughly saturated with the hot oil, salt and pepper.

Pour over a tomato sauce made by boiling tomatoes with the "bouquet" as given in rule for tomato cookery. Serve with grated cheese and a sprinkle of saffron flowers if you like.

Potatoes Scalloped With Herbs

Chop fine, fresh marjoram, savory, chives, thyme, parsley, lovage, about a cupful in all, but not too much lovage.

Butter a baking dish. Put in a layer of peeled raw potatoes sliced very thin, a layer of celery cut in small pieces. Dot with butter, paprika, salt. Sprinkle with the fresh-chopped herb leaves. Make another layer like this and pour over all half milk and water. Bake very slowly, covering it first, and when the potatoes are nearly "done" add a thin layer of buttered crumbs, return to the oven and brown slightly.

Scalloped Oysters

Butter a shallow glass baking dish. Put in a layer of oysters, sprinkle over this a mixture of chopped fennel, basil, parsley, chives, paprika, salt. The next layer may be whole mushrooms which have been lightly browned in butter, *or* boiled Jerusalem artichokes, *or* celery cut in small pieces.

The next layer should be oysters over which the mixed chopped herbs are sprinkled with dry buttered crumbs. Pour over all a thin cream sauce made with the oyster liquor and cream or top milk. Bake about $3/4$ of an hour in moderate oven.

This is a most delicious and "different" dish.

Herb Cheese

One pound of cottage cheese. Blend with this, mixing thoroughly, ½ cupful mixed chopped herbs, paprika, salt, juice of half a lemon, ¼ teaspoon mustard, a drop or two of Worcestershire sauce, mayonnaise, or thick cream to a "spreading" consistency. The herbs used are those of individual preference, but sage and chives in this mixture are important.

Rosemary Biscuit

Two cups of bread flour, into which are cut 1/3 cup shortening and 1/4 cup finely chopped rosemary leaves. (If the dried herb is used, the leaves must be soaked in hot milk till soft.) Add 1 cup milk, 3 teaspoons baking powder, salt, and 1/3 cup sugar. Roll lightly, cut in blocks, and bake carefully. These should be browned, but not hard. Other herbs may be used in the dough, as sage biscuit with chicken and turkey, chopped parsley and cress biscuit with meat and fish salads.

Muffins With Sweet Chervil or With Rose Geranium Leaves

Chop the soft, leafy parts finely and add the grated peel of an orange to a raised dough which has been prepared for tea biscuit. Mould by hand and make a cut in the center of each muffin. Press into this dough a lump of sugar which has been rolled in the chopped herb and orange mixture. Brush melted butter over the tops, raise again, and bake lightly. These muffins have the most indefinable flavor imaginable.

Sesame Oatmeals

2 cups rolled or Quaker oats
2½ cups boiling water
2/3 cup crisco
½ teaspoon salt
1 tablespoon sugar

Cook oats in boiling water 3 minutes. Add sugar and salt. Add crisco unmelted and let melt in hot porridge. Roll while hot, using only flour enough to roll thin. Sprinkle with sesame seed, roll, and bake in a hot oven (350°). Cut into small squares or triangles. These look and taste something like "Educators" and will keep indefinitely in glass jars. The cook may prefer to mix the sesame seed with the oatmeal before rolling. *(Courtesy Mrs. Bancroft Davis.)*

Cumin Cookies

These were served by the hostess at a meeting of the Federated Garden Clubs of New Hampshire and so many were the demands for its recipe that I give it here.

One-half cup butter, ¾ teaspoon baking powder, pinch salt, 1 cup sugar, 1½ cups flour.

Cream sugar and butter, add beaten egg. Sift flour, baking powder, and salt, and work into the egg mixture. Cook slowly 2 teaspoons cumin seed in 1 tablespoon water for 5 minutes. Add to mixture. Chill, roll, cut in thin slices, sprinkle with sugar and bake (375°) for 12 minutes. Sixty cookies. *(Courtesy Mrs. Julius Zieget.)*

Saffron Cake

The dried and crumbled flowers of safflower are used more often than the true saffron. A small amount is mixed with any butter cake batter or stirred lightly into the white frosting of sponge cake. It is bright gold in color.

Jellies

Currant jelly is made in the usual way and just before it reaches the "rolling boil," a large handful of spearmint leaves and tops are stirred in and crushed with a spoon. They should not remain longer than three minutes. The jelly is then strained into glasses.

Lemon thyme may be substituted for mint, and both these useful and delicious jellies used in flavoring gravies for boiled meats.

Apple jelly is made of Porter apples in the usual way, but flavored at the very end of boiling period with leaves of sweet geranium, balm or apple mint. Either strain into glasses or leave a leaf in each tumbler for decoration.

Peach jam is much more flavorsome if the pulp is boiled with lemon thyme a few minutes before pouring into the glasses.

I have tasted sage jelly made with Certo. It is good.

A highly flavored jelly, with more tang, to serve with a roast can be made by using sweet marjoram, either green or dried, with a certo or apple base. A lemon, skin and pulp, may be boiled until soft with the juice.

Mint Sauce for Grapefruit

Mix ½ cup of mint tips, packed hard, ½ cup of water, and 1 cup of sugar or honey and boil for about five minutes. Add green coloring if desired. When cool add to fruit and let stand two or three hours. If you prefer a sweeter sauce add more sugar, but vary the flavor with different kinds of mint—spearmint, peppermint, orange, apple and pineapple mint.

Candied Lovage Root, or Sweet Flag

Dig root in the fall, when it is fully "ripe." Clean, scrape, and cut crosswise into sections. Boil gently in water to cover for several hours, changing several times. Pour off the water and crystallize the root sections in a boiling sugar syrup, made by adding 2 cups of granulated sugar to ½ cup of water. Boil to 300°. When sections of the root are clear, lift them carefully and spread separately on butter paper. Granulated sugar may be sifted over the pieces. This is an old rule of the Shakers. Leave in a cool oven until thoroughly dry, and pack in boxes.

Candied elecampane root was prepared likewise. It made a soothing cough tablet, well known in Shaker times.

Horehound Candy

One ounce of dried horehound herb, leaf, stem, flowers, steeped for 2 minutes in 2½ quarts of boiling water. Strain and squeeze through cheesecloth and allow the tea to settle. Then decant. Add: 3 cups of granulated sugar, 1 teaspoon cream of tartar to 2 cups of horehound tea.

Boil to 240°, add teaspoonful of butter and continue boiling without stirring until the temperature reaches 312°. Remove from the fire and add 1 teaspoonful lemon juice. Pour into a buttered pan. When cool, block in squares, roll in confectioners' sugar, and pack in airtight jars.

A handful of fresh lemon thyme added to the steeping brew of horehound leaves gives a more medicinal flavor, pleasantly soothing to sore throats.

Candied Mint Leaves

Pick the largest, prettiest leaves of spearmint or peppermint. They must be dry and clean. Dip both sides in the slightly-whipped white of eggs or brush over with a solution of gum arabic. Holding by the stem, coat both sides of the leaves immediately with granulated sugar and lay carefully on waxed paper. Allow to dry thoroughly before packing in boxes. To hasten drying, turn the leaves once. They will keep for a year green and sugary.

Sugared Flowers

These are lovely confections for nibbling. Salvage the five-petaled blue corollas of borage, for instance, before they fall and treat the same as mint leaves. The egg may be applied with a camel-hair brush. Rose petals, violets, and cowslip flowers are also used with the spicy fringed petals of the gilly or clove pink.

Garnishing With Herbs

Whoever lives with an herb garden soon realizes that parsley is by no means the only "garnish herb." Young burnet leaves and chervil are equally interesting. Marigold flowers, borage, and nasturtium buds *(Trapaeolum)* take the place of capers.

Tiny nosegays of herbs, pleasant to feel and smell, are fastened in little holders to the side of the finger bowl. Frequently, burnet, geranium leaves and lemon verbena are floated in the bowl.

Young leaves of clary are dipped in batter which has been sweetened with orange and sugar, fried, and used as a garnish for roasts.

Menus

Now and again a request for menus comes in from Garden Clubs when some meal, in which herb cookery predominates, is to be served on their "herb-garden day."

Breakfast

Orange juice with tips of orange mint
Herb omelet
Bacon fried with tender tips of garden thyme
Muffins
(Before baking sprinkle lightly with sesame or poppy seed)
Coffee

Lunch

Tomato-juice cocktail made with herbs and served with potato chips which have been spread with cream cheese and sage
Scalloped oysters with herbs
or with sausages fried with fresh sage leaves
Green salad with honey-and-herb dressing
Hot rosemary biscuit
Fruit cup with chopped pineapple mint
Tea—iced or hot—with lemon thyme or peppermint

Dinner

Cranberry cocktail with herbs
Sesame oatmeals
Roast pork with herb stuffing
Scalloped potatoes with herbs
Green string beans (sprinkled *lightly* with marjoram)
Jellied tomato salad made with tarragon vinegar
and chopped basil
Peppermint ice, served with sponge cake which has been
baked on rose geranium leaves

For afternoon tea there are any number of interesting and tasty herb combinations, spicy spreads on crackers, sandwich fillings, and hot herb teas with seed cakes.

CHAPTER XIII
CHECK LIST OF HERBS FOR MODERN GARDENS*

THIS is a list of the so-called herb genera and their species which might find representation in every modern herb garden.

The comparatively few species recorded, although I am by no means familiar with all, are included in the hope that for other gardeners equally interested in adding to their herb gardens, it will prove, though far from complete, useful as a check list to which with increasing interest many species or varieties may be added.

Species and varieties listed are generally adapted to New England. Some are more or less hardy according to rigors of the climate. A few are tender herbs, but valuable additions to the greenhouse or window garden.

All lists are compiled from catalogues, both American and European. In addition, information has been obtained from various private gardens and commercial nurseries. No name is listed that has not had horticultural recognition. Authorities are not given.

Synonyms are frequent and often are as confusing to the botanist as to the amateur. Two varieties of the mountain thyme, *Thymus serpyllum*, differently named, may be one and the same, but vary in character with soil and climatic conditions. Varietal importance has been listed only as such, and too much credence cannot be placed in the stability of characteristics.

Even though doubtful, a few species have been recorded for the research-minded. From these investigators records of observation and experience will be welcomed.

---

*Nomenclature based on "Standardized Plant Names," 2nd edition. (See *Herb Garden Plants.*) By H. P. Kelsey and W. A. Dayton. Horace McFarland, Publisher.

Already the growing interest in herb gardening during the last few years has resulted in a greatly increased number of fragrants or aromatics in the herb garden of today.

Everyone who has attempted to obtain exact information in regard to these plants, and to learn the distinction between actual species and horticultural varieties, knows that the nomenclature in some groups is in great confusion. Faced with this difficulty, many comparative studies in the Gray Herbarium of Harvard University, Cambridge, Massachusetts, have been made in an attempt to bring as much certainty as possible to the following list. It is realized that this is only a sincere beginning in what must be a long and difficult task. But to anyone really interested in these plants this difficulty should be only a stimulus to further investigation, which will add zest to the cultivation of the living plants in the garden.

I would not add to these species much dissertation upon their individual merits for by their growers some are loved, some scorned. "Liking" is individual. The weedy little *Achillea annua* is to some a loved fragrant in the herb garden, and lamium, the garden pest of aristocratic herb borders, is cobbler's bench of a childhood garden laden with memories.

Any species of particular herb interest is marked (*).

Achillea ageratifolia	Greek yarrow.
A. ageratifolia aizoon	Leaves mostly entire.
A. ageratum	Sweet maudlin. Yellow flowers, pretty, fragrant.
A. alpina	White flowers.
A. argentea	Silvery yarrow.
A. filipendulina	Showy yellow flowers. Coarse fernlike foliage.
A. ligustica	Lovage yarrow. Used as an herb in the making of a cordial. Flowers white.
*A. millefolium	Yarrow, milfoil. A common weed with white flower heads.

A. millefolium rubrum	Red yarrow.
A. moschata	Musk milfoil. White flowers, musky fragrance.
A. nana	Silvery—low rock-garden herb, white flowers, aromatic flavoring of chartreuse.
A. ptarmica	Sneezewort. Has semi-double white flowers. An old-fashioned favorite. Several horticultural varieties.
A. santolinoides	Woolly leaves, white flowers. Called by Stephen Hamblin "False Lavender Cotton Yarrow." A low, gray border herb.
A. sibirica	A low plant with shining foliage and rose-colored flowers.
A. tomentosa	Woolly yarrow. A carpeter. Yellow flower heads on foot-high stems.
A. umbellata	A charming little gray yarrow from Greece with mats of small white flowers.

The achilleas or yarrows are easily cultivated perennials, interesting and spicily aromatic. Most of them have fernlike decorative leaves and white, rose-colored or yellow flowers, which give the garden color from summer to late fall. They are strong aromatic herbs, the whole top of which is used medicinally. Of more than a hundred species of the temperate zones, many are too weedy to be included in the herb garden of even the most enthusiastic collector. Some are tall perennials, good for open garden situations. Others are dwarf carpeters best included in the rock garden. All are sun-loving plants which will withstand drought, wind, and the poorest of soil conditions.

They may be propagated by seed, root division and cuttings. Best soil for the achilleas is light, well-drained and gravelly.

Culpepper, who has much to say about the medicinal virtues of the milfoils, tells of the use of sweet milfoil or maudlin with costmary for sweet washing water.

Several species are used as a substitute for grass or ground covers.

Ajuga chamaepitys	Yellow bugle.
A. ciliare	Downy. Does not creep. Flowers in full blue spike. A showy pink variety is now offered in the nurseries.
A. genevensis	Tufted bugle weed. Does not spread.
A. reptans	Bugle weed, carpenter's weed, sicklewort. A low creeping perennial with early blue flowers; a good carpeter for bare, shady spots.
A. reptans varieties	Several color varieties with variegated leaves—bronze, white and yellow.

These hardy herbaceous perennial herbs, originally from the temperate regions of Europe, are becoming popular as ground covers for shady places under shrubbery. Their heavy, short spikes of deep blue blossoms make a mass of lovely color in early spring.

Seeds, if obtained, may be sown in the open in any kind of soil. Plants are propagated from rooting runners. The "spreaders," however, must be held severely in check unless we need them for cover where no grass can grow.

Allium ascalonicum	Pot herb. Shallot. May be raised from seeds, thinning out to three to four inches. Its "cloves" used like onions for the most delicate flavor.
A. cepa	Pot herb. Onion.
A. cepa viviparum	Top onion with bulbels borne with flowers on tall stems.
A. flavum	An interesting allium for the flower garden with drooping yellow flowers.
A. karataviense	Lilac-blue flowers, blossoming in July.

A. moly	Yellow garlic. Round heads of yellow flowers.
A. neapolitanum	Daffodil garlic. White flowers with green stamens. Ornamental.
A. porrum	Pot herb. Leek. Blanched swollen bases of the leaves are used in salads and sauces.
A. pyrenaicum	A pretty, low edging herb with silvery-purple florets.
A. sativum	Pot herb. Garlic. Greenish-white flowers and a compound bulb, the parts of which are called cloves.
*A. schoenoprasum	Chives. Small perennial onionlike plants with dark green grasslike foliage growing from the thickly clustered little bulbs. Flowers in purple heads. Propagated by seed and division of the bulbous clump. Leaves used for delicate onion flavoring in cookery.
A. schoenoprasum sibiricum	Siberian chive. Larger leaves with less flavor.
A. scorodoprasum	Rocambole. Cultivated for its bulbs which are more delicately flavored than garlic.

Leek, garlic and shallot are bulbous edible herbs. Their herbal history is cloaked in superstition and magic, even to the moment when Satan fled the garden of Eden. Garlic sprang up from the spot where he placed his right foot, and onion from that place his left foot touched.

The genus includes interesting garden species, many of them with lovely color, which are not only good for edging, but valuable for the consummation of color schemes in the herbaceous border.

The accepted mode of cultivation is to sow seeds in rich, friable soil and keep the plants well weeded and free from grass. The thickened or bulbous roots are easily divided.

Anchusa azurea   Italian bugloss. A perennial with bright blue flowers.

*A. officinalis   Alkanet, dyer's bugloss. Hairy herbs with coarse leaves, blue flowers in June; a true biennial. More weedy than *A. azurea*.

There are about forty species of Anchusa from the Old World. They are lovely herbs for extra colors and interest in the herb garden.

Sow seed very early in frames and transplant into common soil. A red dye is made from the root and used to stain woods.

*Anethum graveolens Dill, "Meeting Seed." A famous annual culinary herb. Yellow flowers and soft, feathery leaves.

A. officinale   Sulfur root.

This is one of our best known and popular herbs. There seem to be about one hundred species according to Willis, scattered over the temperate regions of the globe.

Seeds should be sown in good soil where the plants are to remain, with plenty of room for a good second crop, which will appear from self-seeding in the same season. It is well to gather the seeds, which ripen early, by collecting and drying the whole flower head, when they may be gently rubbed out and stored in cloth sacks.

Oil is distilled from the whole plant.

*Angelica archangelica   Garden or officinal angelica. A handsome biennial, which may be made perennial by cutting, after blossoming, the tall, handsome stalks. Flowers greenish-white in large umbels.

A. atropurpurea   Purple-stemmed angelica or masterwort. Greenish flowers; roots said to be poisonous when fresh.

A. sylvestris   Wild angelica. White flowers.

A. curtisi   Wild in eastern United States.

It is interesting to realize that twenty species of the genus *Angelica* are inhabitants of the temperate zones of the earth. Once the garden angelica was found in every herb garden, grown for its manifold uses, but now is imported from Thuringia and Saxony where its culture is associated with legend and folklore dating back to very ancient times. A sweetmeat of commercial importance is still made of the stems, candied and crystallized, and the young tips are used to flavor jams. From its root and seeds an oil is distilled which flavors chartreuse, vermouth, bitters and herbal beverages. This oil also was used in delicate perfumery—Chypre.

Seeds do not germinate easily and before ripening they are attacked by a plant louse which destroys the germ of the seed. Constant spraying of the flower umbel from earliest stages with pyrethrum insecticide is necessary. If allowed to self sow around the old plant they will make good seedlings the first year, which the next season will grow into six-foot stalks with huge divided leaves and are most decorative additions of the herb gardens. They like partial shade, and damp soil, fairly rich.†

Anthemis cinerea	A spreading plant. Daisylike flowers, soft, gray foliage.
A. macedonica	Dwarf, white flowers, pretty in borders.
A. montana	Purplish white.
A. nobilis	Roman chamomile. White-rayed flowers, yellow centers. A lovely little medicinally aromatic plant with fernlike leaves. Dried flowers used in a hair-wash lotion. To make a perennial ground cover, flowering stalks must be kept cut.
A. nobilis florepleno	Double flowers, usually seedless (but save all that show "good doubling").

†See *The Herbarist*, 1937, Publication Herb Society of America, "Angelica Archangelica, The Great Umbellifer," Edgar Anderson.

A. nobilis grandiflora	Large, sometimes yellow flowers.
A. tinctoria	Golden marguerite or yellow chamomile. A good border plant, but a "spreader." Flowers all summer and fall. Varieties are cream color. Perry's variety has large flowers, pale yellow, like marguerite.

Both perennial and annual chamomiles seed readily in the poorest soil at any time of the year and are easily transplanted. The central yellow cone of the chamomile flower is the medicinal part of the plant. The showy horticultural varieties with their lovely yellow and white ray flowers are not accepted in herbal therapy.

Of the hundred or more European species and varieties originally known in Europe, several besides common chamomile are now added to the herb garden for their beauty alone. But no garden is complete without *Anthemis nobilis*, the real chamomile, the virtues of which have been recognized since centuries before Christ when the Egyptians worshipped this little herb beyond all others. (See *Matricaria*). Probably chamomile tea was then used for a sedative and for fevers as now in gentle herbal therapy. Some authors speak of the plant's great curative power over other herbs and bid us use this "plant physician" as they so designate chamomile, to prevent undue withering in our gardens.

*Anthriscus cerefolium	Chervil. Annual or biennial with a carrotlike root and fernlike leaves which turn a pinkish bronze. Fragile white bloom.

There are ten species of *Anthriscus* native in the Eastern hemisphere but this is the only one of herbal importance. The whole plant is a good pot herb, but the leaves are famous for garnishing and seasoning.

Seed early in good loam not too rich and cultivate as carrots. Shade desirable.

CHECK LIST OF HERBS FOR MODERN GARDENS

Amoracia lapathifolium	Horse radish. A coarse-leaved perennial herb with whitish flowers. The thick, sharply aromatic roots of horse radish are well known. The herb grows best in good garden soil. The roots are dug late in the fall and ground, either fresh or dried, for sauces.
*Artemisia abrotanum	Southernwood or old man. A woody shrub with finely-cut, fragrant leaves. (An interesting variety of this species sometimes appears in old gardens.)
*A. absinthium	Wormwood. Flavor used in cordials.
A. albula	Silver king. Tall, decorative.
A. annua	An old-fashioned annual, sometimes called "ambrosia." Four feet, soft, feathery foliage, very fragrant.
A. arborescens	A woody shrub, with finely-cut greenish foliage.
A. arbuscula	Low sagebrush. A silvery, low shrub, gray-leaved, about two feet.
A. austriaca	Silver-gray, soft foliage.
A. californica	California sagebrush. Flowers, yellow-red. Sometimes called "old man," a low, woody bush, and an early medicinal of Colonial Spanish settlers.
A. camphorata	A three-foot shrub, useful in borders, camphor-scented.
*A. dracunculus	Tarragon. The only entire-leaved artemisia. Anise-flavored leaves used in salad.†
A. filifolia	Leaves linear, three-parted.
A. frigida	Fringed wormwood. This species did not appear in America till 1826. Very lovely soft, silvery foliage.

---

†See "Tarragons Cultivated and Wild," Edgar Anderson, *Herbarist*, Publication Herb Society of America, 1936.

A. glacialis	A yellow-flowered alpine, gray, woolly foliage.
A. longifolia	Very white and woolly, simple, entire leaves.
A. ludoviciana	Much like *A. purshiana*, but green on the upper surface of the leaves.
A. mutellina	An alpine form, low, silvery, finely-cut foliage.
A. pontica	Roman wormwood. One to two feet. Feathery foliage. Spreads rapidly.
A. procera	A shrub much like southernwood but taller and more finely cut.
A. purshiana	Cudweed. Decorated, undivided leaves, very white and tomentose.
A. rupestris	A silky-leaved, dwarf rock plant, with nodding yellow flower heads.
A. sacrorum	Russian wormwood. Annual, greenish-white.
A. sacrorum viridis	Summer fir.
A. stelleriana	Beach wormwood or "old woman." Dusty miller is another common name.* Common on sandy beaches, where it makes spreading white patches. Silver-white divided leaves, yellow flowers.
A. tridentata	Sagebrush of western prairies.
A. vulgaris	The common mugwort, which may easily become a garden pest, but if confined and not allowed to seed, it can be used as a tall seven-foot herb for background or in tubs on porches. It has fragrant foliage, green above, silver tomentose beneath. Turns reddish-purple in the fall.

---

*The "Dusty Miller," well-known gray Victorian border plant, often seen in plantings with geraniums, belongs to another genus *Senecio leucostachys*, or *S. acanthifolius* (*Cineraria maritima*). Also "Dusty Miller" is a common name for *Centaurea cineraria*.

A. vulgaris lactiflora	White mugwort. A tall, decorative border herb. Introduced by Wilson from China.

Artemisia is the famous "Armoise" of the French, the mugwort and wormwood of old England and the Colonies. The genus has over two hundred perennial and a few annual species, and they inhabit all parts of our Northern hemisphere. Some are tiny alpines and some are weedy shrubs of the wayside, farmyard, and western prairie. Their leaves are always decorative, for the most part finely cut and silvery green. The flowers except for a few species are not conspicuous, with yellow, greenish and white heads.

Propagation varies slightly with the different species. Tarragon roots must be divided early in the season.

Artemisias need poor, sandy or gravelly soil and the plants thrive best in warmth and sunlight. Pruning of the shrubby, woody varieties should be done cautiously, never cutting off all the new growth at once. Before the leaves of the shrubby artemisias, as southernwood, are out in March the old growth may be cut from the center of the bush. This method of pruning keeps the growth tidy and vigorous. These cuttings should never be wasted, because they will make good plants if "slipped" in water or wet sand.

The artemisias always have been and still are valuable medicinal herbs. Likewise their leaves, stems and flowers are used for perfume and for culinary flavor.

Asperula odorata	Sweet woodruff. Little herbs with creeping roots, whorled leaves, and small white flower heads which bloom very early in the spring. The entire plant is fragrant when dried.
A. orientalis	Blue woodruff. A dainty blue annual, a foot high.
A. cynanchica	A trailing pink-flowered woodruff which does best in sandy soil.

A. hexaphylla	Misty woodruff. Small white flowers, like babysbreath. Stays in bloom for several weeks.
A. longiflora	Low-growing thick mats with pale pink tubular flowers.
A. tinctoria	Dyer's weed. A pest with white flowers and red roots used for dye.

There are, of this genus, more than seventy species originally from southern Europe. They belong to the RUBIACEAE or MADDER family with the coffee shrub, the cinchona tree, from which we obtain quinine, the bedstraws and the little bluet of spring pasture lands. The woodruffs like moist, shady places with good soil.

Seeds should be fresh, sown early in frames and transplanted where they will have room to self-sow, for this is the best of ground covers. Propagates also by root division.

A. odorata loves a place, perhaps, under the elder in the herb garden, where it gets only the shifting sunlight. Even when left under the snow all winter the dried brown stems and leaves smell as sweet as new-mown hay.

This herb is used in white wine and the German "May Drink."

Borago officinalis	Borage. Rough-stemmed and leafy annuals with lovely racemes of blue flowers.
B. officinalis alba	White borage.
B. laxiflora	Seeds and reseeds until freezing. Dwarf; a good rock plant, perennial.

If seed is planted early enough, the self-sowing of old plants makes a new bed which blossoms until after frost.

There are only three species in Mediterranean Europe, and all are largely cultivated for bee feeding. Pliny tells us how the leaves and flowers of borage were used in wine to impart to them its invigoration, to "make men and women merry and drive away all sadness, dulness and melancholy!"

Brassica chinensis	Pot herb. Chinese cabbage, Pakchoi.
B. hirta	White mustard.
B. nigra	Black mustard. An erect annual to three feet or more in height with smaller flowers than the white mustard. The powdered seed of black mustard is that which makes the almost universally-used condiment, mustard.
B. oleracea	Wild cabbage.
B. oleracea acephala	Kale.
B. oleracea botrytis	Cauliflower.
B. oleracea capitata	Cabbage.
B. oleracea gemmifera	Brussel sprouts.
B. oleracea gonglylodes	Kolrabi.
B. oleracea italica	Broccoli.
B. oleracea pekinensis	Celery cabbage, petsai.
B. rapa	Turnip.

Although the mustards have escaped as annoying weeds, if kept in check their yellow flowers are decorative in the herb garden where these old herbs properly belong. Improved varieties are offered as "greens" by the nurseries.

Calamintha (calamint)	For the species once included in this genus see *Satureia*.
*Carthamus tinctorius	Safflower, dyer's saffron and false saffron.

A few seed firms list a supply of seeds of this tall annual belonging to the composite family. Carthamus came to England from Egypt, in 1557. It is easy to grow and is an interesting herb. The orange flowers are made into yellow dye, one use of which is a rouge pomade. They also take the place of true saffron for flavoring. Sow the seed where it is to grow, and thin, but preferably do not transplant. *Crocus sativus*, true saffron, is an iris. *Colchicum autumnale*, meadow saffron, is a lily. *Carthamus tinctorius*, safflower, is a composite.

Carum carvi   Caraway. Biennial, about two feet high, with finely-cut leaves and white flowers in umbels, blossoming in July and August.

Sow seed very early in the spring, thin, do not transplant, and keep weeded. So used are we to caraway seed in our cakes and breads, liqueurs and confectionery, that it is not generally known that the slender tap root of this herb is most deliciously edible.

It grows in most parts of the northern hemisphere, but except in our herb gardens, the United States knows only its seeds as a commercial import from Holland.

If these biennials are given a light winter cover, they will bloom earlier the next spring and have thicker, better foliage.

Chrysanthemum cinerariaefolium   Dalmatian pyrethrum. A silvery-leaved perennial with shining daisylike flowers which make insect powder.

C. majus   Camphor plant. Blooms in spring. White-rayed flower heads. Has strong camphor smell.

C. majus tanacetoides   Sweet Mary. Costmary. Alecost, Patagonian mint. Has rayless yellow flower heads. An interesting perennial grown for its long, mint-flavored leaves. The plant is a great spreader and needs to be confined.

C. parthenium   Feverfew.

Cochlearia   Scurvy grass. Annual with smooth, round leaves and pretty white flowers. It looks almost like candytuft.
officinalis

It is mentioned frequently in the old medical herbals as a scurvy-preventing herb and in the old days sailors on their long sea voyages obtained their vitamins from scurvy-grass ale.

*Colchicum   Meadow saffron. Rose-colored dainty lilies which appear in fall long after the broad green leaves, which come in very early spring, have disappeared.
autumnale

A clump of *Colchicum autumnale*† will increase in size in any garden of light soil for many years. Bulbs are planted in the spring or fall, or seeds may be sown in very fine soil. These will, in five years, give large flowering plants. The root and the seed make the famous homœpathic remedy for rheumatism.

*Coriandrum   Coriander. Annual; tender herb, growing about two feet high. Flowers in pinkish umbels.
sativum

There are several species, but coriander is the only one ever seen in the herb garden. The seeds are strong smelling and have a vile taste when fresh, but become fragrant and pleasant when dried.

Seeds germinate readily when the ground is warm and successive plantings should be made, for the life span of this annual is short. Thin, but do not transplant. Self-sown seeds make tall, sturdy and decorative plants.

*Crocus sativus   True saffron. Lovely fall crocuses of pale lavender with grasslike leaves.

There is a pretty story of how the saffron bulb came, centuries ago, to England in a Crusader's staff and of its popularity with the court ladies as a dye for their hair. King

Henry forbade this use because it deprived him of this greatly-esteemed herb which he enjoyed as a flavoring in his food.

The saffron crocus is one of the most welcome additions to the fall herb garden. The bulb should be planted in light, loamy soil, with a protective winter covering. The flowers appear in early September, and the long, yellow stigmas of the pistils hang out over the pale corolla, giving the chief color to a bed of this herb. These frail little yellow stigmas alone are the only part of the whole plant which is dried, and because of their peculiar pungency find important use in medicine, coloring and cookery.

Needless to say that it takes many thousands to make a pound of saffron. Small wonder, then, that the cost is often prohibitive, and we depend upon the annual saffron, *Carthamus tinctorius*, as an adulterant.

If the bulbs are planted between clumps of mountain thyme a pretty effect is obtained. The saffron flowers are tall enough to push above the shining leaves of the thyme and storms cannot then beat them down into the dirt, bedraggling and tearing their petals. Also thyme is a good winter cover for the bulbs, which need this or some other protection. The only danger in planting bulbous herbs under ground covers of thyme, savories or nepetas is that the mat-like growth of the latter becomes too thick to allow the bulb's growing tip to push through, and then we may find a thwarted little flower or a decayed bulb as belated warning. But naturally this difficulty is obviated by lifting and thinning out the thymes each spring when at the same time we may separate and plant the bulbous offsets.

It takes at least three years to get flowering plants of *Crocus sativus* from seed.

*Cuminum cyminum Cumin. An interesting little annual with pale pink flowers and soft foliage.

---

†See *Herbarist*, 1939, "Colchicine," Mabel L. Ruttle.

The classical herbalists have much to say of this herb, a native of Egypt, which has been known and used since Bible times. It is seldom seen now in any garden and the seed is not easily obtained, except in the European and Asiatic countries. Here, as in our Southern states, although caraway has become more popular, cumin is still sprinkled on cakes and bread. The seeds should be sown early indoors and transplanted into a warm, sunny spot in good soil. This process is by no means always successful, for the seedlings do not thrive in our cold nights and windy spring days.

Only the seed, which is somewhat larger than caraway, is used in cooking for spice, medicine and in veterinary practice.

Foeniculum piperitum — Sicilian fennel. Carosella. Grown for the young edible shoots.

*F. vulgare — Sweet or officinal fennel. Perennial with tall, shining stems, feathery leaves and yellow flowers.

*F. vulgare dulce — Florence fennel or finochio. Annual; short stems, swollen at the bases. Should be treated as a biennial or annual.

There are only three species of the genus *Foeniculum*, all natives of the Mediterranean countries, though they have now spread or been carried into most parts of the world. They are easily raised from seed, sown early in rich soil and transplanted. Stems, leaves and seeds are used as a vegetable, flavoring and medicine. The seeds of sweet fennel are greatly esteemed as a sweetmeat, though as one of the "meeting seeds" which Mrs. Earle describes in "Old Time Gardens," they seem today not so necessary.

One of the prettiest vegetable exhibits I ever saw was that of an Italian grower. It was a great display outlined with the dried, fragrant bunches of Florence fennel.

Hyssopus aristatus — Latest flowering of all species. Heavy, full-flowered racemes.

*H. officinalis	Hyssop. Blue flowers.
H. officinalis albus	White hyssop.
H. officinalis grandiflorus	Sometimes shows double flowers.
H. officinalis ruber	Pink hyssop.

A valuable herb for borders and for general use in any kind of a garden. It is a smooth, dark green, woody perennial which does not lose its color until March. The blue racemes of flowers appear from June until long after frost. Seed should be sown in frames in March. Transplant the inch-high plants into good soil, well limed, about six inches apart. The older plants are apt to grow straggling, but shrubby young ones may be kept ready to fill in the places by propagation of cuttings and root divisions. The foliage is better in partial shade. Leaves, stems and flowers are used in medicinal teas, and some vegetable cookery.

Lamium album	White archangel. Has a long season of showy white bloom.
L. amplexicaule	Henbit. A low annual weed with lavender flowers often seen in cultivated ground.
L. galeobdolon	Yellow archangel. Larger flowers, pale yellow with reddish spots.
L. maculatum	Spotted dead nettle. White and green foliage.
L. purpureum	Purple dead nettle. Darker foliage.

Lamiums, once "simples" of consequence in medicine, now are used for their attractive leaf and flower color in ground covers for damp, shaded places. They look much like our common nettles but, as their name indicates, they do not sting.

Lavandula dentata	Jagged lavender. Tender greenhouse plant.

*L. officinalis or L. vera	Sweet lavender. The true English lavender of all herb gardens and the earliest to bloom. Pale blue flowers.
L. officinalis alba	White flowered lavender.
L. officinalis atropurpurea	
L. officinalis compacta nana	Dwarf French lavender.
L. pedunculata	Narrow-leaved shrub, deep purple, large flowers. Not always hardy.
L. pinnata	Gray, finely-cut foliage, late blooming, blue flowers. Like L. dentata, these are valuable additions to the midsummer herb garden which will carry the lavender's blooming period from spring to fall.
L. spica	Probably a variety of L. officinalis, but not so hardy. It has broader leaves and fewer flowers on the spike, and blooms later in the season.
L. stoechas	French lavender. Odor unpleasant, and plant not hardy.

The lavenders are perennial, shrubby plants, strongly aromatic, which have been great favorites in gardens of all sorts from time immemorial. Folklore, superstition and tradition are woven into the history of this herb, through ages before the Christian era.

The flowers are lavender, purple or white, the leaves are often gray and hoary, and the whole plant is used for medicine and perfume. The blossoming season extends from June to late summer. The best soil is light, mixed with plaster rubble in a warm, airy spot in the sunny corner of an herb garden, or on a wall around it. The shrubs last about three years, when they are likely to grow straggly, so that the beds are best renewed each year. Winter-killing is a complaint made frequently about lavender in New England. Prune as you may need the clippings for bouquets, potpourri and garlands, from spring to Christmas, and never waste a leaf or blossom.

The seed must be fresh and sown early in fine, sterile soil in flats or frames. Keep moist and transplant the seedlings into suitable soil about four inches apart.

Lepidium sativum Cress, peppergrass. Quick-growing spicy annual. Invaluable for salads and for a garnish. Sow seeds early.

Levisticum officinale Old English lovage or garden lovage. Smooth, tall perennial with large, shining, compound leaves and greenish-yellow flowers.

This herb was much in use before the fourteenth century, when its seeds, leaves and roots were used in medicine. The odor is pleasant and not overpowering, and the flavor that of licorice.

Seed may be sown in early spring, but to insure germination, which is uncertain at best, they must be fresh. The old plants will live for many years, and may be propagated by root division in the spring.

Majorana hortensis Sweet or knotted marjoram; perennial but must be cultivated as an annual in the north. Soft-foliaged bushy little herbs very aromatic with flowers in curious hop-like inflorescence, white.

M. onites Pot marjoram. Perennial with larger flowers than *M. hortensis*. Introduced in 1759. For description of genus, see page 169 under *Origanum*.

Marrubium astracanicum More like *M. vulgare*, but with blue flowers and more wrinkled leaves.
M. candidissimum Often with yellowish foliage.
M. catariaefolium Rare. Very woolly, flowers pink.
M. serbineum A broader, rounder woolly leaf. Rather a nice ground cover.

M. vulgare Horehound. Hoary, perennial, shrubby plants with white flowers in bristly whorls.

There are thirty species of *Marrubium* in Europe, North Africa and temperate Asia, and we have by no means exhausted their possibilities as good introductions into our herb gardens, for their gray foliage is an interesting note in midsummer.

Horehound is raised very easily and it is well to plant a goodly patch for cutting when in bloom. Dried slowly, the leaves, stems and flowers make a healthful tea which is not only used in curing feverish colds, but is combined with sugar into the famous horehound candy made by the Girl Scouts.

The seed, which should be sown in poor soil very early, germinates slowly. Transplant the seedlings when an inch high, six inches apart, and keep weeded. Cut old stalks to the ground each fall; this will keep the bed thick for several years, but it is always well to start a new bed each spring from self-sown seedlings.

Matricaria chamomilla German chamomile. Medicinal herb; low annual. Makes fine fernlike mats of leaves.

M. eximia Same as *Chrysanthemum parthenium*. The common feverfew of old gardens. A hardy annual.

M. inodora Mayweed. Wild chamomile. A strong-scented but interesting little barnyard weed.

M. tchihatchewi Turfing daisy. A perennial mat-forming plant with white flowers. Suggested as a substitute for grass. Introduced in 1869.

The *Matricarias* make good mats for sunny, gravelly banks. They need little attention, and their cheerful daisylike flowers are compensation for their commonplaceness. Seeds sown in poor soil make the best and most aromatic plants. If used in place of grass the flowers must be cut, but with this self-seeding annual *permanent* ground cover cannot be attained as with the perennial *Anthemis*.

The botanical differences between the German chamomile, *Matricaria* and the true chamomile, *Anthemis*, are minute, though significant enough to warrant a different name for this genus.

An herb-garden enthusiast says that the tea made from the flowers of German chamomile makes a far more soothing herbal brew than that made from the true chamomile, *Anthemis nobilis*.

Melissa officinalis   Lemon balm or sweetbalm. A hardy, herbaceous, perennial herb with spreading root stalks, soft yellow-green foliage and small yellowish-white flowers which bloom all summer. Whole plant tastes and smells like lemons.

M. officinalis aurea   Golden balm. Very fragrant. Leaves more decidedly yellow-green.

There are four European species of *Melissa*, but Colonial gardens, since Pilgrim days, have known and used only the herb first mentioned, known as sweetbalm. The dried leaves, flowers and stems were used by them as a lasting fragrance in potpourri, and invigorating teas.

The seeds germinate slowly and irregularly even though sown in fine soil. They must be kept very damp and transplanted when an inch high into a moist and rich soil. A bed of lemon balm will last for many years, and new plants are easily made by root division. If a few roots are planted in a shallow pot and brought into the house in October, a lovely house plant with trailing fragrant stems is reward indeed.

Mentha aquatica   Watermint. A common "escape" in wet land.

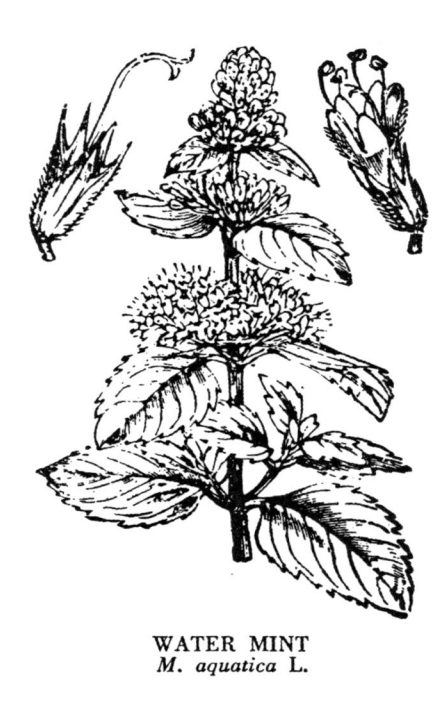

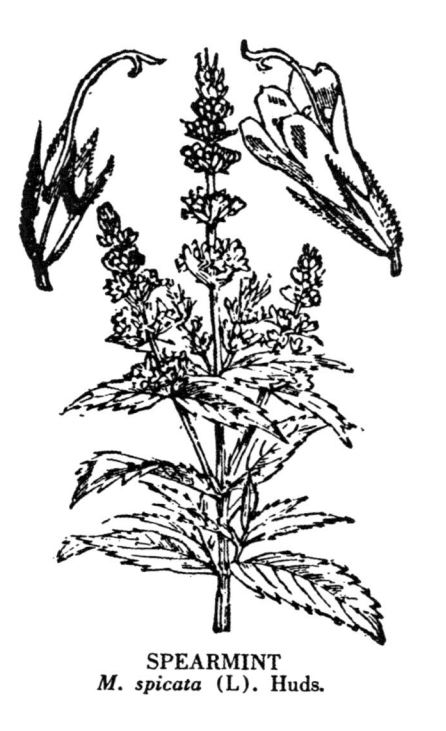

WATER MINT
M. aquatica L.

SPEARMINT
M. spicata (L). Huds.

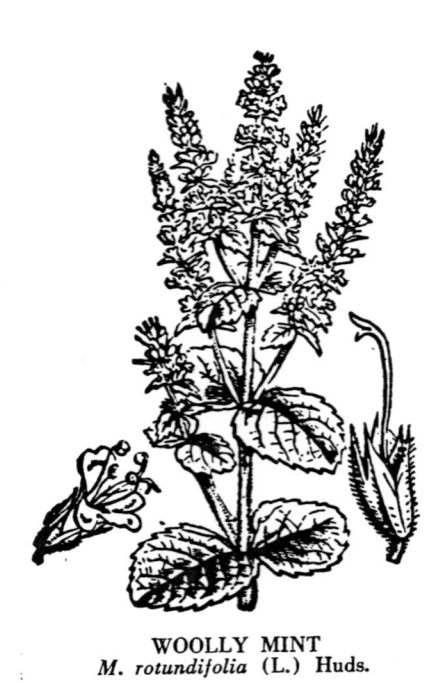

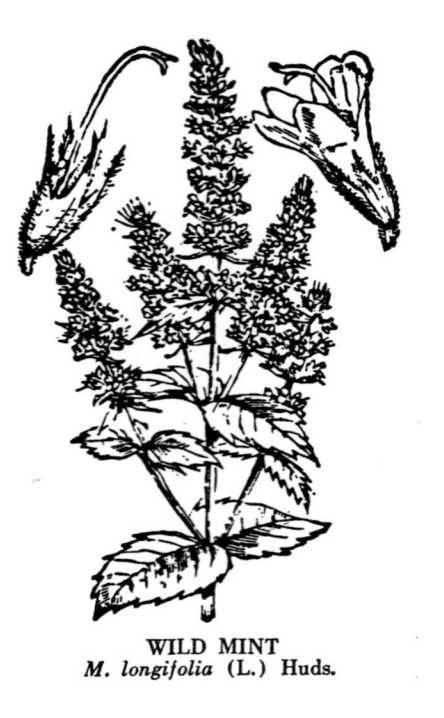

WILD MINT
M. longifolia (L.) Huds.

WOOLLY MINT
M. rotundifolia (L.) Huds.

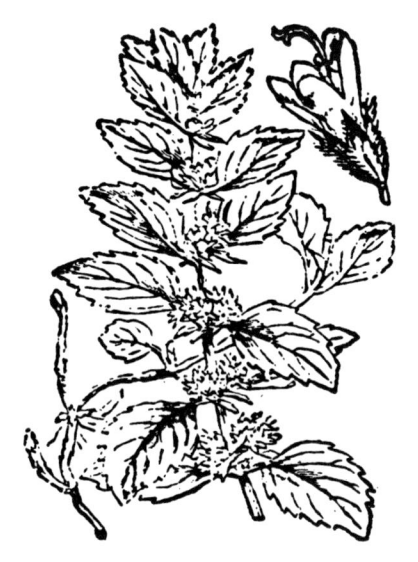

CORNMINT
M. arvensis L.

M. arvensis	Cornmint. Field mint. A coarse plant with many varieties of scent, flavor and names.
M. arvensis canadensis	American wild mint.
M. arvensis piperascens	Japanese peppermint. A stiff-stemmed low-growing variety. Sharply serrate leaves of unpleasant flavor.
M. gentilis	Creeping mint. Golden apple mint.
M. longifolia	European horse mint. Mild flavor.
M. niliaca	Egyptian mint. Tall, gray, woolly.
M. piperita	Wild peppermint.
M. piperita citrata	Bergamot mint. Orange mint.
M. piperita officinalis	Peppermint. The true white or Mitcham peppermint.
M. pulegium	Pennyroyal. Creeping leafy runners with rising stems of blue flowers.
M. requieni	Corsican mint. A strongly-scented plant with tiny leaves and flowers, interesting for crevice planting and shady spots in the rock garden.
M. rotundifolia	Woolly mint. Tall, gray-leaved, spreading, decorative plant with good flavor.
M. spicata	Spearmint. (Probably the same as *M. viridis*.) Hardy herbaceous perennial with creeping root stalks. The whole plant is richly aromatic. Flowers in pale purple spikes. "Commercial spearmint" is a horticultural variety, the true form being useless.
M. spicata crispata	Curly mint. An excellent culinary herb with broad, wrinkled leaves.

NOTE: The author is grateful to Mr. Van Eseltine and Mrs. Ruttle Nebel of the Geneva Experiment Station, New York, for help in preparing this list.

The genus *Mentha* includes forty species of the tropics and temperate zones but specific and varietal importance in this group is most uncertain, and there is a wide field for horticultural and botanical research.

As several of the mints do not produce seed or seed that is certain of germination, propagation is entirely from plant division or cuttings made from the creeping root stocks. Planted in moist soil, these cuttings very quickly grow roots at every node and a pair of leaves. All the mints do well in clay soils and thrive in rich garden loam. They do not like sour soil. If a bed of mint becomes infected with the fungus *Puccinia menthae*, which shows as brown spots on the leaves, the stems must be cut down and burned and a new bed started in another part of the garden; or dust with "Sulfun."

Because the true mints hybridize with each other it is not easy to keep the separate species apart, but it should be the ambition of interested herb growers to grow at least the typical species in the herb garden. †

Micromeria chamissonis	Yerba buena.
M. croatica	A charming little plant with pale lavender flowers.
M. piperella	Peppermint micromeria.
M. rupestris	Prostrate stems with small dark green leaves; flowers, white spotted with purple.
Monarda citriodora	Prairie bergamot. Lemon-scented purple flowers.
M. didyma	Scarlet monarda, Oswego tea, bee balm. Tall, leafy, hardy, herbaceous perennial with scarlet blossoms.
M. didyma alba	White flowers, very dark green foliage.
M. fistulosa	Wild bergamot. Purple flowers.
M. fistulosa alba	Flowers white, lavender tinged.
M. punctata	Spotted flowers.

†See *The Herbarist*, 1938, Publication Herb Society of America, "Some Common Mints and Their Hybrids," Mabel L. Ruttle.

Many varieties are now being introduced into gardens from the Rocky Mountains.

It is interesting to realize that this is one of the very few herbs in modern gardens which has its origin in North America. Monarda was named after the Spanish physician Monardez, who discovered and described this herb in 1656.

It is one of the easiest herbs to raise. Sow the seeds early in rich soil in the open. The plant is a rampant spreader and soon makes tall, big clumps which must be divided. The seeding heads are fragrant and should be saved for potpourri.

NOTE: The true *"Bergamot"* of commerce is the oil extracted from the peel of the fruit of a small citrus tree—*C. Bergamia* (Bailey).

Myrrhis odorata Sweet cicely or myrrh. Perennial herbaceous herb with thick root and fernlike, fragrant leaves. Small white flowers.

There are four European species. The wild sweet cicely of our own woodlands is a different genus although it somewhat resembles the myrrh of the early English gardens.

Sweet cicely seeds itself freely in any kind of soil, but grows best in rich loam under the trees. The plant, seeds and root are used in cookery and medicine.

NOTE: The "myrrh" of commerce is probably the same as the "myrrh" of the Bible. It is the aromatic gum of a tropical tree.

Nepeta cataria Catnip. White or purplish flowers, gray foliage.

N. glechoma or *Glechoma hederacea* Ground ivy, Gill-over-the-ground or ale-hoof. The best of ground covers for shady places with its creeping stems, shining leaves and blue flowers. *Glechoma hederacea variagata* is interesting.

N. macrantha Showy violet flowers. Bushy.

N. mussini Nept. Hardy, herbaceous, low perennial with soft foliage and violet-colored flowers.

N. nervosa	Annual nept. Full light blue heads of flowers. Lanceolate leaves.
N. nervosa alba	White flowers.
N. nuda	A tall, smooth-leaved nept, with attractive flowering stems.
N. wilsoni	A good rock plant with purple flower spikes.

Outside the tropics this genus includes one hundred species. Besides nept, and a few others grown primarily for horticultural purposes, there are two of age-old reputation, catnip and ground ivy.

There are few human beings of recent generations who have not been dosed with catnip tea in feverish colds, and enjoyed its sleep-inducing aroma. Ground-ivy tea dates from Anglo-Saxon days, and is the best of spring tonics.

Aside from growing the plant for its real beauty, set a bed of catnip from which to cut and dry for the cats in winter.

"*If you set it the cats will eat it,
If you sow it, the cats don't know it.*"

The *Nepetas* grow from seed, which ought to be sown, if possible, where the plants are to remain. If they are transplanted to wall gardens or banks, the seedlings must be kept moist until established. After this they will thrive in poorer soil and with less moisture than other mints. For a second blossoming in the fall cut them back in July, and their flowering season will last even through the first frost. Nept does not like lime.

Origanum dictamnus	This is the "Dittany of Crete." Pink flowers. Shrubby, very woolly round leaves, not hardy.
O. heracleoticum	Winter marjoram. White and pink flowers. Introduced in 1640.
O. vulgare	Wild marjoram. Pink flowers. A tall, woody-stemmed garden species. Perennial.

O. vulgare aureum   Golden-leaved marjoram. Seldom seen.

There are thirty European species and each country seems to know and use some favorite variety of marjoram.

Sweet marjoram was a dainty strewing herb for milady's chamber in mediæval England, and its perfume most often included in pomanders and scent bags. Our own Colonials were most familiar with the sweet, or knotted marjoram, for which there were all sorts of uses. Its essence in the culinary bouquet was most delicate, and in potpourri it is indispensable.

All the marjorams like warm, light, dry, chalky soil. Seeds sown in April of any species, both annual and perennial, make good growth and bloom before fall. At this time they should be cut for drying and winter use. Propagate the perennials by root division and pegging down the lax outside stems.

Ocimum basilicum   Sweet green basil. Annual with yellow-green leaves and small white flowers. Fragrant, shrubby plant, a foot and one-half high. Very tender. The French catalogues list several agricultural varieties of this species.

O. basilicum purpureum   Sweet purple basil.

O. crispum   Japanese basil. Called lettuce-leaf basil. Possibly a variety of *O. basilicum*.

O. gratissimum   Tree basil. Listed and described in "New Herbal" by Grieve and Leyell.

O. micranthum   American basil. Grows wild in Florida.

O. minimum   Compact little bushes with small leaves and white flowers.

O. minimum purpureum   Purple basil. A lovely little herb with varying shades of reddish-purple foliage and covered with flowers of the same colors in midsummer.

CHECK LIST OF HERBS FOR MODERN GARDENS 171

O. sanctum   Sacred basil of India. Tulasi. A curiously-scented annual with hairy leaves and stems and pale purple flower spikes.
O. viride   Fever plant.

Forty-five species of *Ocimum* are known in the warm and temperate climates, but in the modern herb garden they are such tender annuals that our enjoyment of them between the spring and fall frosts of New England is short.

Aside from their value as good kitchen herbs they have distinctive beauty, from the little round-topped purple varieties to the ungainly wrinkled leafy plants of the curly basil.

The herb has a hot spicy flavor unequaled for use in tomato cookery of which we are rapidly learning the flavoring secrets from the Mediterranean peoples. In the foreign quarters of our cities, it is not unusual to see, outside the basement doors, pots of growing basil even as in India where it was the herb of family protection.

*Petroselinum crispum   Parsley. Biennial or perennial. Beautiful foliage herbs with dark green curly leaves. Flowers greenish yellow, second season.
P. crispum filicinum   Fern-leaved parsley.
P. crispum neapolitanum   Italian parsley. Celery-leaved parsley. Best for cooking flavor.
P. crispum radicosum   Turnip-rooted parsley. Roots boiled and eaten like parsnips.

There are thirty European species of *Petroselinum* and many varieties have sprung from *P. crispum*, the only one cultivated for commercial purposes. The seeds are slow in germinating and have vitality even when several years old. Thin out in the rows to eight inches in good well-fertilized soil. The plants grow best in partial shade, making crowns of decorative leaves which, beside their beauty in the herb garden, are one of our best herbs for garnishing and flavor. There are many superstitions connected with its cultivation which seem to be combined with the antiquity of this herb.

Transplanting brings ill luck to the gardener, it is said, and that "Parsley seed goes nine times to the devil and comes back" is well believed as we wait for the appearance of the small plants after sowing.

Pimpinella anisum Anise. Hardy perennial with lacy leaves and white flowers. A variety has rose-pink blooms.

Willis records seventy-five species of *Pimpinella* and the garden anise was so loved by Charlemagne that he ordered its planting in all gardens. There is a superstition that anise wards off the Evil Eye. Because "it was used in a spiced cake at the end of a meal by the Romans in Virgil's time to prevent indigestion, a cake which was brought in at the end of a marriage feast, it is perhaps the origin of today's spicy wedding cake." (Grieve and Leyel.)

Sow the seed in very warm soil in May, thin, and keep weeded. It does best in soil not too rich. Dry the flower heads, and rub seeds out carefully.

Rosmarinus officinalis Rosemary. A sweet-scented perennial herb which may grow tall and shrubby with lax, climbing branches. The small blue flowers in the axils of the leaves blossom in April. The leaves are narrow, gray-green, and thickly set upon the stems, with recurved edges. The whole plant is distilled for its valuable aromatic oil and the leaves have some culinary use.

R. officinalis alba White rosemary.
R. officinalis prostratus Lax, prostrate growth making a delightful rock plant.

R. pyramidalis   Possibly a variety of *R. officinalis* with more erect stems and broader, darker green leaves.

Books have been written of the virtues and legends of this herb, which vies with lavender for fame and antiquity. Grieve and Leyel in the "New Herbal" recount the special symbolism attached to this lovely plant. "Not only was it used at weddings, but also at funerals, for decking churches and banqueting halls at festivals, and as incense in religious ceremonies, and in magical spells."

Indoor wintering is safest for New England climates.

The seeds should be sown early indoors in sterile soil and the seedlings transplanted before they are an inch high. The soil should be limed, gravelly, not at all rich.

Propagate by means of cuttings, using large pieces of last year's wood. The outside branches may all be layered in summer by pegging down in the soft earth, covering lightly and keeping wet.

We read of the "gilded rosemary." Who has seen it?

Ruta chalepensis   Fringed rue.
*R. graveolens   Rue. Shrubby herb, about four feet, nearly evergreen in New England. Greenish-yellow flowers.
R. patavina   Dwarf rue. This and fringed rue are modern garden species listed in "Hortus" and should prove interesting if their seeds or plants could be obtained from some European botanic garden.

A shrub of rue is a handsome addition to any garden, because of its shining, blue-green, divided leaves and its curious yellow-green flowers, which cover the shrub in midsummer. To many the scent is not pleasant, but true herb lovers appreciate it.

Rue seeds and reseeds readily in any soil, preferably one well limed. Young plants remain green for a longer period in a New England winter than old shrubs. It transplants well and is easily propagated by layering. Cuttings root quickly. The leaves are used in European countries in salads, and their use here in vegetable cocktails is now popular.

The genus *Rue* is of Mediterranean origin with about five hundred species. *Ruta graveolens* has been cultivated for centuries for its great medicinal and disinfecting qualities.

Because the Four Thieves anointed themselves with a vinegar made of this herb and others, they pillaged and robbed unharmed the plague-infested cottages.

We must remember that it was with euphrasy and rue that Adam's sight was purged by Milton's angel. Aside from its symbolism of repentance, the branches of rue were used as brushes to sprinkle Holy Water before the Mass. It is called the herb-o'-grace, and endowed with great powers of restoring second sight.

Bruised and applied externally, rue leaves are useful in allaying rheumatic pain and headache.

Salvia argentea	Silver sage. Broad, white, woolly leaves.
S. azurea	A lovely blue perennial for the midsummer garden.
S. carduacea	Thistle salvia.
S. farinacea	Grayish foliage and powdery blue flowers.
S. horminum	Annual. Color given by the red-purple bracts of the flowers.
S. horminum violacea	Pink flowers.
S. nemorosa	Violet sage. A beautiful long flowering species.
S. officinalis	Garden sage. A shrubby, gray-leaf perennial which deserves more importance in the flower border.

S. officinalis albiflora	White flowered sage.
S. officinalis Hort.	"Holt's mammoth" var. A more sturdy shrub than the type species, with broader leaves.
S. officinalis purpurascens	Purple garden sage.
S. officinalis rubraflora	Red garden sage.
S. rutilans	Pineapple sage. Tender, fragrant herb for the midsummer garden. Coral-red flowers which blossom late but continue through the winter if the plant is brought inside.
S. sclarea	Clary. Clear eyes. A tall shrub with lovely pinkish-white and blue flowers. The colorful bracts remain through the summer. Large gray leaves. A true biennial.
S. sclarea Turkestanica	White Clary. Pale whitish green bracts.
S. splendens	The common "red sage salvia" of park plantings.

Sage is as valuable an herb for its utilitarian uses as rosemary is for its aesthetic. There are five hundred species of salvia in the tropical and temperate zones. A large number of them have medicinal or culinary value, but garden sage and clary have been known for many centuries in both the old and the new world. The species *officinalis* varies greatly and the old writers describe many varieties, some with red or variegated leaves. There are innumerable legends and quaint beliefs in connection with this herb.

Cur moriatur homo cui Salvia crescit in horto? ("Why should a man die while sage grows in his garden?")

"Sage mitigates grief." There is evidence of this in Pepys' diary, where a little churchyard in England is described with its graves always covered with sage.

The Chinese were fond of sage tea, liking it better than their own garden tea, and as a gentle perspirant it has been a recognized medicine for ages.

The cultivation of all sages is simple. They need limy, gravelly soil. The seeds germinate readily if planted early and transplanted seedlings eight inches apart grow in the same season to good sized bushes. The young stems and leaves are used for cookery, either fresh or dried.

Sanguisorba canadensis	Canadian burnet. Found wild in swamps.
S. minor	Salad burnet. Smaller, more tender leaves.
S. obtusa	Japanese burnet. Showy rose-colored flowers.
S. officinalis	Garden or evergreen burnet. Perennial herbs, hardy herbaceous, with mats of long, compound, crenulate leaves, and tall stems of plumy flowers. Rose colored or white.
S. tenuifolia	Fernlike gray foliage, purplish flowers.

Willis records thirty species in the north temperate zones, but only a few are decoratively interesting to the herb garden. Perhaps not the least value of salad burnet is in its evergreen mats from which the new young leaves grow all winter. They give to our salads and cocktails a distinctive flavor, said by some to resemble cucumbers.

The seeds germinate readily and may be sown very early. When transplanting, it is well to allow a distance of eight inches between the plants, for the spreading crowns are often over a foot in diameter. Propagation is also by root division.

Santolina chamaecyparissus	Lavender cotton or French lavender. (Probably same as *S. incana*.) A low, shrubby perennial with flowers like little yellow knobs. Fine foliage soft gray and fragrant.
S. pinnata	Bright green foliage.

S. tomentosa	A silvery, compact shrub. Excellent as an "accent plant." Larger yellow flower heads.
S. virens	Green santolina. A low, fragrant, green shrub.

Santolina was a favorite edging plant with makers of "knot gardens" and has been returned to gardening favor as an excellent border herb of fragrant, enduring qualities. It is of ornamental growth which should not be checked by reckless pruning. Too much new wood taken off at once causes "bleeding" and subsequent winter-killing.

Some medicinal value is attributed to the whole plant but the Colonials used it as a moth preventive, laying the leafy stems among their clothes. It is also used in potpourri, and in lovely nosegays, with clove pinks and moss roses.

Shrubs of santolina thrive best in well-drained, light soil with warm exposure. Seeding is uncertain. A shrub of lavender cotton will last many, many years. It is easily propagated by pegging down the outside branches into the moist earth. When rooted they may be easily grown by separating from the mother plant.

Satureia acinos	A low growing herb with delicate foliage and purplish flower clusters.
S. alpina	Alpine savory.
S. calamintha	Calamint. Lilac flowered. Once called *Calamintha officinalis*.
S. grandiflora	Sometimes classed as a horticultural variety of *S. calamintha* but with larger, deep purple flowers and coarser growth.
*S. hortensis	Summer savory. Annual, two feet or less. Very fragrant and aromatic.
S. montana	Winter savory. A woody evergreen with white flowers.
S. nepeta	Catnip satureia. Bushy about two feet, flowers pale, fragrant.

S. vulgaris   Basil mint or wildbasil. A weedy herb with whorls of magenta flowers.
S. vulgaris alba   White flowered basil mint.

Willis records well over a hundred species of the genus *Satureia* growing in tropical, subtropical, and warm temperate regions. They are fragrant, mostly low growing herbs which look much like the thymes and nepetas. At the present time the genus *Calamintha* is called *Satureia*. All of the above species except *S. hortensis* are perennial with a liking for a not too rich soil. Seeds may be sown in the open early, but to insure fixity of character in the perennial species, propagation of the plant should be made by division in the spring. More savories are being introduced into our gardens each year and these flower-covered woody little sub-shrubs adapt themselves readily to rock work and edgings.

Summer savory is one of the most useful of the sweet herbs, the young tips and leaves being used both fresh and dried. Its taste is much like that of the winter savory, and both are used in stuffings, soups, and in meat cookery. Fragrance and taste remind us somewhat of marjoram, but the savories are more peppery. The herb is useful when weeding in the garden on a warm summer day for if the leaf is rubbed on bee stings instant relief is afforded.

*Sesamum indicum   Bene, sesame.

This is an annual of the sub-tropics. Several other species in the genus are known, but bene is the one cultivated commercially in the Southern countries where it is still used among the old negroes in medicine, cookery and candy.

Southern seed firms have usually a supply of seed, but, however fresh, its germination is a triumph in any but well-drained soil where there are long, hot days of sun and warm nights. This is not an encouraging prognostication for growing in New England, and it has been an interesting weakling in my own Lexington gardens long enough for me to make its acquaintance only. It is one of the simples used by Hippocrates 400 B.C.

In the classics, several plants are credited with the name sesamum, and heliotrope is called the "great sesamum" by Theophrastus.

Such a profuse nomenclature has grown up around it as almost to obscure this poor little herb. Dioscorides speaks of sesamum, which, however, he says is a tree, and he also gives the name to *ricinus*, the castor-oil bean.

Theophrastus claims that poppy and sesamum seeds had not the "least place" for flavoring, and so the ancients when they wanted to speak of some well-turned phrase or style spoke of it as sprinkled with poppy and sesamum.

Petronius, a Roman voluptuary, at the court of Nero, 60 A.D., says, "They hear honeyed groups of words, sprinkled as it were, with Poppy and Sesamum."

*Sium sisarum Skirret. (See Pot Herbs, page 32.) The foliage is interesting in combination with other herbs. Plant the seeds very early in good loose soil and thin out as you would parsnips. Leave space, for they make large perennial clumps. The roots are boiled and eaten as the early herbalists tell us to "stir up the appetite."

Symphytum asperum Prickly comfrey. Perennial, shrubby herb; often five feet high. Prickly and petioled leaves. Flowers pink and blue in nodding racemes.

*S. officinale Common comfrey. Flowers yellowish, rose purple or white.

S. rubrum A garden variety listed in English catalogue with deep red flowers and said to be a good plant for loamy soil under trees.

There are about fifteen species of this genus and all are most interesting in flower structure, showing clever adaptations for bee pollination. The true comfrey is a rather weedy perennial not often seen now even in the old gardens.

The roots are thickened and when crushed make a gelatinous, healing salve. The leaves were applied to sprains and bruises, and the herb was a great favorite in the early New England gardens as a medicinal simple.

It needs some shade, and thrives under old apple trees.

Teucrium canadense	Woodsage.
*T. chamaedrys	Germander. Little perennial shrubby plants grown for their foliage, which is nearly evergreen. Purple flowers last from July to frost.
T. marum	A low, light gray foliage plant. Purple flowers.
T. massiliense	Purple flowers.
T. polium	Woolly leaves, yellow flowers.
T. pyrenaicum	Flowers pale yellow with lilac markings.

About one hundred species of *Teucrium* are known in the north temperate parts of the world, but *T. chamaedrys* is of chief interest in the herb garden for, though a native of the Orient, it was a precious medical herb of old England. Great was its reputation in herbal therapy as a cure for gout.

In these modern days, however, it is sufficient to use the compact, shrubby little plants of this species as a delightful edging for any garden. The seeds must be planted very early indoors and the plants spaced in transplanting to four inches. Any good garden soil, not too rich, will give good color in leaves and flowers. It is possible to propagate, also, from cuttings taken in early spring.

Thymus alsinoides	Low, pale lavender flowers in July.
T. britannicus	A sturdy, gray, carpeting thyme, round woolly leaves, covered in spring with pink flowers.
T. capitatus †	Showy. Round, rose-colored flower heads.

---

† Headed savory. Is recorded as being in Britain in 1596. It is a seasoning not now mentioned, but was recorded in American gardens as late as 1863.

T. carnosus	Whitish flowers.
T. cimicinus	Red-stem thyme. Low, trailing, fine leaves, large heavy heads of pink flowers in August.
T. erectus	Sturdy little evergreen. Pink flowered.
T. glaber	A thick carpeting thyme almost evergreen. Height about six inches. Pink flowers.
T. herba-barona	Caraway thyme. Slender, trailing stems. Nearly evergreen. Pink flowers, strong scented.
T. hirsutus	Tall. Makes high, thick mats. Hairy flowers, rose color to red.
T. hyemalis	Shrubby, fragrant, dark green. Flowers almost white.
T. jankae	Rose-colored flowers. Makes loose, thick mats.
T. lanicaulis	Long trailing stems, gray and very woolly. Showy pink heads of flowers. June.
T. nitidus	Shrubby, shining, dark green. Pale flowers. July.
T. pectinatus	Very fragrant. Flowers lavender.
T. pyrzewalski	Carpeting thyme. Flowers deep rose.
T. serpyllum	Mother of thyme, mountain thyme. Makes spreading mats of fragrant growth, flowers profusely. Reddish bracts of the flowers persistent. This thyme varies greatly. Is found in all parts of the world.
T. serpyllum albus	White thyme. Bright green. Tiny leaves. Makes thick, close mats which are covered in early spring with drifts of pure white flowers. Ideal for stepping stones.
T. serpyllum argenteus	Silver thyme. Bushy, gray-leaved, shrub, pale pink flowers.

T. serpyllum aureus †	Golden thyme. Low, matted growth. Smooth, dark green leaves, mottled with gold, which become more intense in fall and early spring. It does not bloom profusely.
T. serpyllum azoricus	Slender, narrow, woolly leaves. Thin woody stems. Creeping. Does not winter well nor flower profusely.
T. serpyllum citriodorus	Lemon thyme. This species belongs in every old-fashioned garden. It makes high mats of smooth, green growth from which rise tall stems of pink flowers with colorful persistent reddish bracts. Strong lemon flavor and fragrance.
T. serpyllum citriodorus forma aureus	Embroidered thyme. Thick bushy plants. Dark green leaves mottled or edged with gold.
T. serpyllum comosus	Rose-pink flowers. Low, thick mats. Creeping stems.
T. serpyllum lanuginosus	Woolly thyme. Makes a low, close mat, small, hairy leaves, very gray. It flowers very seldom and does not winter well.
T. serpyllum loveyanus	A good ground cover, thick and high. Blooms profusely.
T. serpyllum micans	Grows in thick "moundy" tufts which are apt to brown and die in the winter. Interesting, not for its flowers, but because it makes vivid green patches between the rocks until late fall.
T. serpyllum montanus	A lovely dark green variety. Smooth, with bright rose-colored flower heads.

† In his leaflet on thymes grown in the Lexington Botanic Gardens, Mr. Stephen Hamblin records this as the thyme spoken of in Mrs. Earle's "Old Time Gardens" and once grown around the base of sundials, for "Time is golden."

T. serpyllum nummularius	High mats, clean green leaves, large heads, showy flowers. Late summer.
T. serpyllum pannonicus	Thick mats of gray leafy stems about two inches deep which are covered with short-stemmed purplish heads of flowers very early in the season.
T. serpyllum pulchellus	This thyme makes thick, leafy, light green mats with close-growing, rose-colored flowers. Invaluable for dry, rocky banks.
T. serpyllum splendens	Smooth green mats, deep red flowers. Very showy.
T. striatus	Makes thick mats. Blooms in midsummer.
T. villosus	Low, soft mats, covered with pink flowers. June.
*T. vulgaris	Garden thyme. Shrubby. Flowers profusely. Almost evergreen. Very aromatic. The species most frequently used for flavoring.
T. vulgaris fragrantissimus	Much like *T. vulgaris,* but grayer, stiffer and more shrubby.
T. zygis	Stiff-stemmed, little thyme with small heads, reddish-purple flowers, very narrow gray leaves. Does not winter well.
T. zygis gracilis	More prostrate than the species. Greener leaves and paler, smaller flower heads.

NOTE: This list of thymes will carry the season of bloom throughout the summer.

The thymes are shrubby, woody plants or low creeping carpeters. Some are tender but others will stand New England weather. The ice and thawing always harm these herbs by heaving them from the ground, thus letting air around the roots. They must be packed firmly back into their beds, or they will winter-kill.

The flowers range from white through all shades of reddish purple, pale lavender, white and pink. In most species the seeds germinate freely and easily. The beds run out in three years and should be renewed by cuttings or layering the stems or starting a new seed bed. The whole plant is dried and used in medicine and flavoring.

Thyme tea is an invigorating tonic for headaches, but aside from its culinary value, thyme is now chiefly used commercially for its volatile oil, thymol, most important as a deodorant and anaesthetic.

Of all the fascinating herb groups for collection and study, the thymes give the keenest horticultural delight. To read of them in their native haunts, the mountains of Crete, the highest crags of the Pyrenees, the slopes of Parnassus, and the sun-baked Smyrnan hillsides is to wonder at their ready adaptability and their enjoyment of our own New England.

The gardener uses them to cover baren banks hopeless for all other vegetation, and they make most welcome additions to rock gardens and perennial borders. Their purple, white and pink blooms rejoice our senses in summer as does their fragrant green foliage in winter.

Thymes make resistant mats between the flagging on which to tread and soft carpets on which to kneel, giving out no protest other than their aromatic, spicy scent. To the discriminating nose, these scents vary. They remind us of peppermint, caraway, lemon, orange, camphor and some dare say that even a garlic odor has been detected or imagined. So he who has a collection of twenty thymes in his herb garden has a daily bouquet of sweet smells, which under the warm summer sun blend into invigorating inspiration.

Thyme flowers and honey are inextricably woven into the literature of the classics. Virgil loved his bees, and no honey in the whole world had the sweet flavor of that made from the wild thyme which still grows today on the slopes of Hymettus.

The charm in color of the thymes is equally intriguing. It may not be vested in the corolla of the flower alone. In some species the long, awned bracts of the calyx take on rosy and lasting deep red hues.

T. membranaceus should become a favorite. A Gray Herbarium specimen shows it to be a lovely little thyme about eight inches high with creamy flowers, long and tubular. The pale pinkish bracts which persist long after the corolla has fallen give permanent flower-like color to this species.

Thymus vulgaris, the garden thyme, is a sturdy little evergreen about ten inches high, fragrant with loose, pale purple flowers which begin to blossom in June. There is a broad-leaved and a narrow-leaved variety from France. Both are equally valuable for flavoring and are the herbs to use in all recipes unless otherwise stated. Sow the seed in open ground in early May. Transplant or thin out the seedlings to four inches apart. A "thick" bed winters best. Do not prune except when needed. This thyme will grow almost anywhere, but loose, sterile well-limed soil makes the most aromatic plants.

The most common carpeting thyme is *T. serpyllum*. It and its many varieties are found in every state in New England, and it is widespread in localities in the United States.

The white thyme, *T. serpyllum albus*, which clings "as tight as its skin" is very lovely indeed and throughout the winter maintains the most vivid green of all the thymes.

T. bracteosus from the Bosnian Mountains is a woody little shrub with narrow, silky leaves, big reddish-purple flower heads. As the specific name implies, these consist of long-awned, persistent bracts which give the color effect rather than the paler flowers.

T. cephalotus from Portugal's high mountains is another showy species with brilliant red bracts at the base of the separate flowerets in large heads. It looks almost like our old friend, self-heal, *Prunella vulgaris*.

I have no doubt that the varietal and specific importance, and perhaps even the authenticity of the thymes listed here may be questioned. The nomenclature of this genus is in hopeless confusion. "Die flora der Mittel Europa," by Gustav Hegi includes a scientific monograph upon this genus, but does not describe the many horticultural varieties which have appeared within the last years. No one treatise on the thymes is adequate for correct identification.

Tanacetum huronense	Large, showy yellow flower heads and coarse, fernlike foliage.
T. vulgare	Tansy, bitter buttons. Perennial. Lovely fernlike leaves, aromatic, with clusters of yellow buttonlike flowers. Tall, shrubby. Now a common weed.
T. vulgare crispum	Is much like the type species, but a smaller plant, with more finely curled leaves.
T. vulgare variegatum	A pretty, striped leaf form.

The genus *Tanacetum* comprises fifty species all growing in the northern hemisphere. Although the escape of the common tansy from Colonial gardens has covered since then many a waste land and ash heap with its sightly green, the herb still deserves a corner somewhere in the modern herb garden.

The records of early New England show no use to which it was not put in those early days of the Colonies. It was a preservative of meat because no flies would light on flesh which had been rubbed with the juice of tansy. Because of its great powers as a vermifuge, it was one of the mediæval strewing herbs. It was used as a medicine, culinary flavor, and a useful embalming herb for the dead. Its growth and spread in any soil is assured if once planted or if seed is sown.

BIBLIOGRAPHY

He who plans an herb garden wisely reads the ancient herbals and many garden books, both old and new. The valued assistance and advice of Miss Dorothy S. Manks, librarian of the Massachusetts Horticultural Society, which has been so cheerfully given me in the compilation of this book, is only the usual courtesy which members of this Society are receiving every day from her and her assistant, Miss Brenda Newton. To all gardeners, their work is a distinct contribution to horticultural research and further study.

These books are in the library of the Massachusetts Horticultural Society. Those marked * may be used only in the reading room.

The art of simpling, by William Coles. Lond., 1657. Repr., Milford, Conn., Mrs. R. E. Clarkson, 1938.

*[Banckes's herbal] an herbal (1525). Brattleboro, Vt., pr. by E. L. Hildreth, 1941.

Book of herbs, by Lady Rosalind Northcote. Lond., Lane, 1903.

*The country house-wives garden, by William Lawson. London, pr. by Anne Griffin, 1637. Facsim. ed., Milford, Conn., Mrs. R. E. Clarkson, 1940.

Culinary herbs and condiments, by Mrs. M. Grieve. N. Y., Harcourt, 1934.

*Culinary herbs, their cultivation, harvesting, curing and uses, by Maurice Grenville Kains. N. Y., Orange Judd co., 1912.

*Delightes for ladies, by Hugh Plat. Lond., 1602. Repr. Herrin, Ill., Trovillion private press, 1939.

*Digitalis, by U. S. Works projects administration of New York City. N. Y., 1939.

*Divers chimicall conclusions concerning the art of distillation, by Hugh Plat. Lond., pr. by Peter Short, 1594. Facsim. ed., Milford, Conn., 1941.

*Flora's dictionary, by a Lady (Mrs. E. W. Wirt). Balt., Lucas, 1855.

Fragrant path, a book about sweet-scented flowers and leaves, by Louise Beebe Wilder. N. Y., Macmillan, 1932.

Garden of herbs; rev. and enl. ed., by Eleanour Sinclair Rohde. Lond., Jenkins, 1926.

Garden of simples, by Martha Bockée Flint. N. Y., Scribner, 1900.

Gardening with herbs for flavor and fragrance, by Helen Morgenthau Fox. N. Y., Macmillan, 1933.

Gardens of Colony and State: gardens and gardeners of the American Colonies and of the Republic before 1840; comp. and ed. for the Garden Club of America by Alice G. B. Lockwood. N. Y., Scribner, 1931-1934.

*Gardens old and new: the country house and its garden environment. Lond., Country life pr.; N. Y., Scribner, 1900-1909. 3 vols.

Gerard's Herball, the essence thereof distilled by Marcus Woodward from the edition of Th. Johnson, 1636. Lond., Howe, 1927.

*Ginseng, by Maurice G. Kains. N. Y., Orange Judd, 1914.

Ginseng and other medicinal plants, by R. R. Harding. Columbus, O., 1913.

Grandmother's herbs and simples, by Anne Mountfort. Damariscotta, Me., the author, 1938.

Green enchantment, by Rosetta E. Clarkson. N. Y., Macmillan, 1940.

Healing herbs of the zodiac, by Ada Muir. Vancouver, B. C., Torch publ. co., 1938.

Herb garden; 2d ed., by Mrs. Frances A. Bardswell. Lond., Black, 1930.

*Herb journal, ed. by Rosetta E. Clarkson, New Rochelle, N. Y., 1936-1939.

Herb-lore for housewives, by C. Romanné-James. Lond., Jenkins, 1938.

Herb primer, by Mrs. G. M. Brown. Topsfield, Mass., Perkins Press, 1939.

Herbal delights, by Hilda Leyel ("Mrs. C. F. Leyel"). Boston, Houghton, 1938.

The Herbalist, by J. E. Meyer. Hammond, Ind., Indiana Botanic Gardens, 1934.

*Herbals, their origin and evolution, a chapter in the history of botany, 1470-1670; new ed. rewritten and enl., by Agnes Arber. Camb. (Eng.) Univ. pr., 1938.

The Herbarist, 1935—, published by the Herb Society of America, Horticultural Hall, Boston, Mass.

Herbs for urbans — and suburbans, by Katherine van der Veer. N. Y., Loker Raley, 1938.

Herbs, salads and seasonings, by X. Marcel Boulestin. Lond., Heinemann, 1930.

Herbs, their culture and uses, by Mrs. R. E. Clarkson. N. Y., Macmillan, 1942.

Home and garden: notes and thoughts, practical and critical, of work in both, by Gertrude Jekyll. Lond., Longmans, 1900. (See Chap. 15—"The making of pot-pourri.")

*Lexington Leaflets of the Lexington Botanic Garden, Mass., Apr. 11, 1931—(Various issues devoted to herbs).

Magic fragrance, by Rosetta E. Clarkson. New Rochelle, N. Y., 1937 (repr. of the first 12 issues of the Herb Journal).

Magic gardens, by Rosetta E. Clarkson. N. Y., Macmillan, 1939.

Magic in herbs, by Leonie de Sounin. N. Y., Barrows, 1941.

Magic of herbs, a modern book of secrets, by Mrs. C. F. Leyel. Lond., Cape, 1926.

Mediæval gardens: "flowery medes" and other arrangements of herbs, flowers and shrubs grown in the Middle Ages, with some account of Tudor, Elizabethan and Stuart gardens, by Sir Frank Crisp; ed. by C. C. Paterson. Lond., Lane, 1924. 2 vols.

Modern herbal: the medicinal, culinary, cosmetic and economic properties, cultivation and folklore of herbs, grasses, fungi, shrubs and trees, by Mrs. Maude Grieve. Lond., Cape; N. Y., Harcourt, 1931. 2 vols.

*New principles of gardening, by Batty Langley. Lond., 1728.

Old English gardening books, by Eleanour Sinclair Rohde. Lond., Longmans, 1922.

Old roses, by Mrs. Frederick Love Keays. N. Y., Macmillan, 1935.

Old time gardens newly set forth, by Alice Morse Earle. N. Y., Macmillan, 1931.

Old time herbs for northern gardens, by Minnie Watson Kamm. Boston, Little Brown, 1938.

Olden time beverages, by Alice Earle Hyde, Brooklyn, N. Y.

*Paradisi in sole paradisus terrestris, by Jon Parkinson: faithfully reprinted from the edition of 1629. Lond., Methuen, 1904.

Plantes et santé; 2e ed. by Henry Correvon. Paris, Delachaux et Niestlé, 1922.

Plants used as curatives by certain southeastern tribes, by Lyda Averill Taylor. Cambridge, Mass., Botanical museum of Harvard University, 1940.

Poisonous plants of the United States, by Walter Conrad Muenscher. N. Y., Macmillan, 1939.

*Resources of southern fields and forests; new ed., by Francis P. Porcher. Charleston, S. C., 1869.

Rose recipes, by Eleanour Sinclair Rohde. Lond., Routledge, 1939.

Sachets and seeds, by Rosetta E. Clarkson. Milford, Conn.,

1938. (Repr. of the second 12 issues of the Herb Journal.)

Salads and herbs, by Cora, Rose and Bob Brown. Phila., Lippincott, 1938.

Scent of flowers and leaves, its purpose and relation to man, by Frank A. Hampton. Lond., Dulau, 1925.

The Still-House. Boston, Herb Society of America, Horticultural Hall, 1935.

Sun-dials and roses of yesterday, by Alice Morse Earle. N. Y., Macmillan, 1902.

*Sweet-scented flowers and fragrant leaves, interesting associations gathered from many sources, with notes on their history and utility, by Donald McDonald. Lond., Samson Low, 1895.

Text-book of pharmacognosy; 4th ed. rev. and enl. by Heber W. Youngken. Phila., Blakiston's, 1936.

*The toilet of flora. Lond., pr. for J. Murray, 1779. Repr. Milford, Conn., Mrs. R. E. Clarkson, 1939.

Vegetable cultivation and cookery, by Eleanour Sinclair Rohde. Lond., Medici, 1938.

What to do with herbs, by Mary Cable Dennis. N. Y., Dutton, 1939.

The Williamsburg art of cookery, compiled by Mrs. Helen Bullock. Williamsburg, Va., pr. for Colonial Williamsburg, inc., 1938.

HERBALS

*The Badianus manuscript, an Aztec herbal of 1552. Baltimore, Johns Hopkins press, 1940.

*Five hundred points of good husbandry, by Thomas Tusser, with an introduction by Sir Walter Scott and a benediction by Rudyard Kipling incorporated in a foreword by E. V. Lucas. Lond., Tregaskis, 1931.

*The Herball, or Generall historie of plantes, by John Gerard. Imprinted at London by John Norton, 1597.

*Paradisi in sole paradisus terrestris; or A Garden of all sorts of pleasant flowers, by Jon Parkinson. Lond., printed by Humphrey Lownes, 1629.

*Stirpium historiae pemptades sex sive libri XXX, by Rembertus Dodonaeus. Antwerpiae, ex officina Ch. Plantini, 1583.

Index

Achillea, 142-4
—— millefolium, 32, 70
Aconite, 27, 42
Aconitum napellus, 27
Acorus calamus, 67
Actaea alba, 68
—— rubra, 68
Adiantum pedatum, 69
Agastache, 20, 103
Agrimonia striata, 67
Agrimony, 67
Ajuga, 29, 144
Alecost, 154
Aletris farinosa, 68
Alexanders, 33
Alkanet, 27
Allium, 35, 144-5
Althaea rosea, 30
—— officinalis, 30
Alum root, 68
Ambrosia, 27
Anchusa, 27, 146
Anethum graveolens, 29, 146
Angelica, 42, 146-7
Anise, 27, 172
Annual herbs, 94
Anthemis, 29, 147-8
Anthriscus cerefolium, 148
Aralia nudicaulis, 68
Archangel, 158
Arisaema tryphyllum, 68
Armoracia lapathifolia, 149
Arrachs, 33
Artemisia, 43, 149-51
Asarum canadense, 69
Asperula, 31, 151-2

Balm, 42, 162
Balmony, 64
Baneberry, red, 68
——, white, 68
Basil, 27, 170-71
Bee garden, 18

Bellis, 42
Bene, 178-9
Bergamot, 167-8
Betonica officinalis, 27
Betony, 27, 29, 70
——, wood, 27, 70
——, woolly, 27
Bibliography, 187-92
Birth root, 68
Blitum, 34
Bloodroot, 68
Boneset, 66
Borage family, 73
Borago, 152
Bowman's root, 66
Box, 42, 53
Brassica, 153
Broom buds, 69
Bugle, 29, 144
Bugloss, viper's, 32
Burnet, 176
Butterfly weed, 20
Buxus sempervirens, 53

Calamint, 29
Calamintha officinalis, 29, 153
Calendula officinalis, 31, 43
Camphor plant, 154
Caltha palustris, 66
Campanula rapunuloides, 35
——, rapunculus, 35
Caraway, 29, 154
Cardamine pratensis, 43
Cardinal flower, 68
Carnation, 42
Carthamus tinctorius, 153, 156
Carum carvi, 29, 154
Catnip, 29
Ceanothus americanus, 70
Cedronella, 103
Celandine, 68
——, lesser, 69
Celery, 33

Centaurea, 29, 66
Centaurium umbellatum, 29, 66
Centaury, 29, 66
Centory, 29
Centum aurum, 66
Centranthus ruber, 31
Chamomile, 29, 42
Chaste tree, 42
Chaucer daisy, 42
Checkerberry, 69
Check lists, herbs, 141
Chelidonium majus, 68
Chelone, 64
Chenopodiaceae, 76
Chenopodium Bonus Henricus, 34
———, botrys, 27
Chervil, 148
Chicory, 29
Chives, 145
Chimaphila umbellata, 69
Chrysanthemum, 29, 154
Cicely, sweet, 31, 68, 168
Cichorium intybus, 29
Cimicifuga racemosa, 68
City Herb Garden, 27
Clary, 29
Cloister gardens, 26
Club mosses, 68
Cochlearia, 155
Cohosh, black, 68
Colchicine, 29
Colchicum, 29
———, autumnale, 29, 155
Colic root, 68
Colonial garden, 47
Coltsfoot, 66
———, sweet, 53
Comfrey, 29, 179
Commercial, Growing, 104
Composite family, 75
Convallaria majalis, 32
Cooking with herbs, 120
Coptis trifolia, 66
Coriander, 29, 155
Coriandrum sativum, 29, 155
Costmary, 29, 154
Cottage industry, 118
Cotton, lavender, 176
Cough remedy, 116
Cowslip, 29, 43

Cress, 29, 35
Crevices, herbs for, 98
Crithmum maritimum, 36
Crocus, saffron, 31
——— sativus, 31, 155
Crow-bell, 43
Crow-flowers, 43
Crown imperial, 43
Cruciferae, 77
Cuckoo buds, 43
Cuckoo flowers, 43
Culture, general, 88
Culver's physic, 66
Cumin, 29, 156-7
Cuminum cyminum, 29, 156-7
Cunila origanoides, 30
Curing herbs, 106
Cytisus scoparius, 69

Daffodil, 43
Deacon Goodale Farm, 50
Devon Gardens, 24
Dian's bud, 43
Dianthus caryophyllus, 30
Dictamnus albus, 29
Dicentra canadensis, 69
Digitalis purpurea, 30
Dill, 29, 43
Dipsacus fullonum, 70
Dittany, 29, 169
Doctrine of Signatures, 79
Drosera, 67
Drying herbs, 106

Echium vulgare, 32
Edging, herbs for, 100
Eglantine, 43
Elecampane, 30
Enclosures, 24
Endive, 33
Eruca, 34
Erythraea centaurium, 29
Eupatorium perfoliatum, 66
———, purpureum, 66
Evergreen herbs, 96
Exedra, 25

Families, herb, 71
Fennel, 30, 43, 157
Fern, 43
———, maidenhair, 69

INDEX 195

——, rock, 69
Feverfew, 30, 154
Flag, blue, 64
——, sweet, 67
——, yellow, 67
Foeniculum, 30, 157
Foxglove, 30, 43
Fraxinella, 29
Furniture, garden, 25

Galega officinalis, 66
Gardens, bee, 18
——, cloister, 26
——, colonial, 47
——, Devon, 24
——, knot, 41
——, ladder, 49
——, mediæval, 22
——, pot herb, 32
——, renaissance, 36
——, Shakespeare, 42
——, Still-Room, 44
——, Stuart, 40
——, Tudor, 36
——, wild, 62
Garlic, 34, 35, 145
Gaultheria procumbens, 69
Genista tinctoria, 32, 70
Geranium robertianum, 30
Geraniums, sweet-scented, 58
Germander, 30, 180
Gillenia trifoliata, 66
Gill-over-the-ground, 52, 168
Gilly-flower, 30, 43
Ginger, wild, 69
Ginseng, 69, 85
Goldenrod, anise, 68
Golden seal, 68
Goldthread, 66
Good King Henry, 34
Goosefoot family, 76
Grape flower, 60
Grass, scurvy, 155
Ground covers, 96
Ground nut, 69

Harebell, 43
Heartsease, 43
Hedeoma pulegioides, 70
Hellebore, green, 66

Henbit, 158
Hepatica, triloba, 69
Herb, families and genera, 71
——, menus, 139
——, recipes, 127-39
Herb o' grace, 66
Herb Robert, 30
Herbe de St. Pierre, 36
Herbs before 1700, 59
Heuchera americana, 68
Hollyhock, 30
Honeysuckle, 30, 43
——, English, 56
——, Italian, 56
Hop, 55
Horehound, 30, 161
Horse-radish, 77, 149
Hortus Inclusus, 25
Hydrastis canadensis, 68
Hyssop, 30, 43, 157-8
Hyssopus, 30, 157-8

Incense, 114
Inula, helenium, 30
Iris, 30
——, florentina, 30
——, pallida, 30
——, pseudacorus, 30, 67
——, versicolor, 64
Isatis tinctoria, 32
Ivy, 43

Jack in the pulpit, 68
Joe Pye Weed, 66

Knot gardens, 41

Labiatae, 76
Ladder garden, 49
Lady-smock, 43
Lamium, 158
Larkspur, 43
Lavandula, 30, 158-60
Lavender, 30, 43, 158-60
——, French, 176
Ledum groenlandicum, 66
Leguminosae, 78
Lepidium sativum, 160
Lettuce, 33
Levisticum officinale, 160
Lilium candidum, 30

——, canadense, 68
Lily, 30, 43
——, Canada, 68
——, Madonna, 30, 55
Lily family, 76
Lippia, citriodora, 103
Lobelia, blue, 68
——, cardinalis, 68
——, siphilitica, 68
Long-purples, 43
Lonicera caprifolium, 56
——, periclymenum, 30, 56
Loosestrife, purple, 67
Lotions, 115
Lousewort, 70
Lovage, wild, 33
Lychnis, floscuculi, 43
Lycopodium, 68
Lythrum salicaria, 67

Marigold, 31, 43
——, marsh, 66
Marjoram, 43, 160, 169-70
Marrubium, 30, 160-61
Mary bud, winking, 43
Matricaria, 29, 30, 161-2
May apple, 68
Meadowsweet, 69
Medicinal herbs, 27, 81
Mediæval gardens, 22
Melissa officinalis, 162
Mentha, 162-67
Micromeria, 167
Milkweed, orange, 20
Mint, 43, 53, 162-67
——, family, 76
——, mountain, 70
——, Patagonian, 154
——, pool, 26
Mitchella repens, 69
Mitrewort, false, 69
Monarda, 167-8
Moon, influence of, 91
Mosquito bush, 103
Mount Vernon, 56
Mugwort, 31, 151
Mulberry tree, 43
Mullein, 31
Mustard, 34, 153
——, family, 77

Myrrhis odorata, 31, 168
Myrtis communis, 103
Myrtle, 103

Native herbs, 64
Nepeta, 29, 168-9
Nettle, dead, 158
Nymphaea odorata, 32, 67

Ocimum basilicum, 27, 170-71
Onion, 43, 144
Orachs, 33
Orchis, 43
Origanum, 29, 169-70
Osmorhiza claytoni, 68
——, longistylis, 68
Oxlip, 31, 43

Paeonia officinalis, 31
Panax schinseng, 69
——, trifolium, 69
Pansy, 43
Papaver somniferum, 31
Parsley, 43, 171-72
——, family, 77
Partridge berry, 69
Pea family, 78
Pedicularis canadensis, 29, 70
Pelargonium, 58, 59
Pennyroyal, wild, 70
Peony, 31, 43
Perennial herbs, propagation of, 94
Perfumes, 114
Periwinkle, 31
Petasites, 53
Petroselinum, 171-72
Pilewort, 69
Pimpinella anisum, 27, 172
Pink, 43
——, clove, 30
Pipsissewa, 69
Pitcher plant, 67
Plants, colonial, after 1700, 60
Pleurisy root, 20
Podophyllum peltatum, 68
Polemonium caeruleum, 31
Polypodium vulgare, 69
Polypody, 69
Pomanders, 114

INDEX

Pool, mint, 26
Poppy, 31, 43
Porch boxes, herbs for, 100
Pot herbs, 32
Potpourri, 114
Primrose, 31, 43
Primula elatior, 31
—— veris, 29
—— vulgaris, 31
Prince's pine, 69
Propagation, perennial herbs, 94
Punch, herb, 127
Pycnanthemum, 70
Pyrethrum, Dalmatian, 154
Pyrola rotundifolia, 69
Pyroly, 69

Ragged robin, 43
Rampion, 35
Ranunculaceae, 86
Ranunculus ficaria, 69
Renaissance gardens, 36
Rocambole, 35
Rocket, 34
Rosa, 31, 58
Rose family, 78
Rosemary, 31, 172-3
Roses, old, 57, 60
Rosmarinus officinalis, 31, 172-3
Rue, 31, 43, 173-4
——, American goat's, 64
——, goat's, 66
Rumex scutatus, 34
Ruta, 31, 173-4

Safflower, 153
Saffron, annual, 156
——, crocus, 31
——, meadow, 29, 155
——, true, 155-6
Sage, 174-6
Salads, herb, 101
Salvia, officinalis, 174-6
——, sclarea, 29
Samphire, 36, 43
Sanguinaria canadensis, 68
Sanguisorba, 176
Santolina, 176-7
Sarracenia purpurea, 67

Sarsaparilla, wild, 68
Satureia, 177-8
Savory, 43, 177-8
Scilla nonscripta, 43
Scrophulariaceae, 86
Seed sowing, 89
Sesamum indicum, 178-9
Shakers, 81
Shakespeare gardens, 42
Shallot, 35
Shin leaf, 69
Shrubs, before 1700, 60
Signatures, Doctrine of, 79
Simpler's joy, 64
Sium sisarum, 179
Skirrets, 34, 179
Smallage, 33
Snakeroot, black, 68
——, white, 68
Snapdragon, 43
Snuffs, 117
Solanaceae, 86
Solidago odora, 68
Sorrel, 34
Southernwood, 43, 149
Speedwell, 31
Spiraea salicifolia, 69
——, tomentosa, 70
Squaw berry, 69
Squirrel corn, 69
Stachys lanata, 27
——, officinalis, 27
St. Barbara's herb, 34
Steeple bush, 70
Still-Room garden, 44
Stock, 43
Strawberry blite, 34
Stuart gardens, 40, 41, 43
Sundew, 67
Superstitions, 113, 172
Sweetbriar, 31, 43
Sweet Mary, 154
Sweet William, 43
Symbolism, 109-13
Symphytum, 29, 179-80

Tanacetum, 70, 186
Tansy, 70
Tarragon, 149
Teasel, 70

INDEX

Tea, Labrador, 66
——, New Jersey, 70
Teas, herb, 123
Tender herbs, 103
Tephrosia virginiana, 64
Teucrium, 30, 180
Thistle, 43
Thoroughwort, 66
Thyme, 31, 43, 180-86
——, wheel of, 48
Thymus, 180-86
Tiarella cordifolia, 69
Transplanting seedlings, 91
Trillium, 68
Tudor gardens, 36
Turtle head, 64
Tussilago farfara, 66
Tussie mussies, 110

Umbelliferae, 77
Uses of an herb garden, 109
Uses of herbs in garden planting, 96

Valerian, 31
Valeriana, officinalis, 31
Valley lily, 32
Veratrum viride, 66
Verbascum thapsus, 31
Verbena hastata, 64
——, lemon, 103
——, officinalis, 31, 66
Veronica officinalis, 31
Veronicastrum virginica, 66
Vervain, 31
——, blue, 64
Vinca, major, 31
——, minor, 31
Viola odorata, 32
Violet, 32, 43
Vinegar, aromatic, 117
——, herb, for cooking, 126
Vitex agnus-castus, 42

Waterlily, 32, 67
Wattle fences, 25
Wheel of thyme, 48
Wild gardens, 62
Window gardens, herbs for, 100
Wintergreen, 69
Winter protection, 93
Woad, waxen, 32, 70
——, wild, 32
Woodruff, 151-2
——, sweet, 31, 53
Woodsage, 180
Wormwood, 43, 149-50

Yarb patch, 50
Yarrow, 32, 70, 142-4
Yerba buena, 167